DENTAL IMPLANTS

Fundamental and Advanced
Laboratory Technology

Robert Winkelman, CDT
Kenneth Orth, CDT

exclusive distribution worldwide

M Wolfe

Exclusive distribution worldwide,
except Spain:

M Wolfe

Mosby-Year Book Europe Limited

Lynton House
7-12 Tavistock Square
LONDON - WC1H 9LB
England

ISBN: 0.7234.2040.8

A CIP catalogue record for this book is available from the British Library

© Espaxs, S.A. Publicaciones Médicas, 1994
Rosselló, 132
08036 - Barcelona
(Spain)

Printed in Spain

FOREWORD

DENTAL IMPLANTS: Fundamental and Advanced Laboratory Technology, is a landmark text in the field of dental technology. With the popularization of osseointegrated implants in the dental profession following the Toronto conference in 1982, dental implantology has increased significantly. The specialties of prosthodontics, periodontics and oral surgery, in addition to advanced general practices, have incorporated osseointegrated implants into the daily treatment of patients with missing teeth. This increased use created significant change and more creative demands on dental technicians. The construction of the implant-supported prosthesis requires special knowledge and cooperation between the technician, the clinical practitioner, and the patient.

Because the technology of osseointegrated implant-supported prosthodontics is significantly different from that of traditional crown and bridge fixed prostheses, this textbook holds a very special place, not only in academic dentistry, but in a more practical sense in its ability to provide dental technicians with greater insight and knowledge, and assist them in building precision implant-supported bridges.

In reviewing the history and rational of osseointegrated implants in the first chapter, Mr. Orth and Mr. Winkelman point out the fundamental premise of success for osseointegration. The biomechanical union of the implant fixture to living bone requires very precise surgical manipulation. The continued success of this treatment then depends on the expert technical skills required in building the bone-anchored bridge. For this reason more than ever before, the dental technician truly becomes an integral part of the treatment team and has a direct responsibility for the successful prognosis for every patient treated with osseointegrated implants.

In the early 1980's, a small handful of specialists in North America embarked on a program of using osseointegrated implants for the restoration of edentulous and partially edentulous patients. Mr. Orth and Mr. Winkelman became an integral part of that early team concept and worked closely with the pioneers of osseointegration. As clinical experience and knowledge grew, so too did the body of information in the dental laboratory. The standard restoration originally initiated by Professor Brånemark and his Swedish research colleagues for the complete mandibular arch reconstruction is well described in the third chapter. Mastering the fundamentals of this reconstruction then led to the expansion of technology in it's relationship to other implant manufacturers and systems, and also expanded the horizons of ingenious techniques to compensate for complex problems inevitably present with difficult clinical reconstructions.

Porcelain technology involves special considerations for the implant prosthesis supported by osseointegrated fixtures. The technical difficulties related to porcelain shrinkage and warpage of frameworks is logarithmically multiplied in the ability to fit the implants. The forgiveness of the periodontal membrane present in traditional fixed bridgework is not available with osseointegrated implants. This places a more exciting and demanding burden on the dental technician to produce exquisitely fitting castings both before and after the application of porcelain.

The chapter on porcelain application is very helpful, especially with the insights gained from framework distortion experience when large castings receive multiple firings. Dealing with this problem through an evolution of methods resulted in a successful procedure for maintaining precision fit of the implant gold superstructure.

Additional chapters on combination fixed and removable implant-supported prostheses, including the slant lock retention system, serve as an excellent guide to the construction of this prosthesis.

The inclusion of experimental frameworks, such as the carbon fiber-reinforced acrylic bridge described in Chapter 8, provides excellent information on possible alternative forms of prosthesis construction. Although this technology differs significantly from traditional standards, the information is valuable for any technician who wants to stay abreast of current research endeavors.

Some of the very best information in the text is related to the single tooth replacement system. The Brånemark System fixture is used as the implant fixture for the single tooth. A variety of substructures and abutments, including the UCLA system, can be adapted to this implant for successful function as well as esthetic results.

Esthetic problem solving described in Chapter 9 truly shows the ingenuity that dental technicians possess, creating the illusion of natural teeth supported by the osseointegrated implants. Resolving esthetic problems leads very nicely into the guidelines of general problem solving and trouble shooting outlined in Chapter 10.

I take a great deal of personal pride in the enormous effort put forth by Ken Orth and Bob Winkelman in their production of this textbook. I have worked closely with both of these certified dental technicians since the inception of osseointegration in North America and have watched the exciting growth of technology in this field. Ken Orth and Bob Winkelman have indeed proven themselves leaders in osseointegrated implant dental technology and I compliment them on their courage in undertaking this monumental task and for the production of this text book.

Thomas J. Balshi, DDS, FACP
Prosthodontics Intermedica
Institute For Facial Esthetics
Fort Washington, Pennsylvania

CONTENTS

The Brånemark System is a registered trademark of Nobelpharma AB.
Core-Vent is a registered trademark of the Core-Vent Corporation.
The Slant-Lock Retention System is a product of the Evelyn Co. Inc., Tulsa, OK.

NOTICE

Dentistry is an ever-changing science. As new research and clinical experience broaden our knowledge, changes in treatment are required. The editors and the publisher of this work have made every effort to ensure that the procedures herein are accurate and in accord with the standards accepted at the time of publication.

Chapter 1

History and Rationale

In 1952 P.I. Brånemark began scientific studies and later clinical research which led to his observation of the process of osseointegration. Osseointegration is the direct structural and functional union of ordered living bone to the surfaces of a load carrying implant.[1] This scientific breakthrough is rapidly changing the practice of implant prosthetics in dentistry today. It has equally effected dental laboratory procedures related to the fabrication of implant-supported prostheses. The introduction of osseointegration to North America in the early 1980's has created new challenges and opportunities for dental technicians. Totally new concepts of prosthesis design continue to evolve. Structural engineering principles must be combined with artistic skills to build an accurately fitting, durable and esthetic prosthesis.

Although Brånemark's research and clinical applications initially focused on the completely edentulous arch,[1] Balshi,[2] Sullivan[3] and Jemt[4] have successfully applied these same principles to the restoration of the partially edentulous patient. Many partially edentulous patients reject the concept of restoring healthy teeth with conventional fixed or removable prostheses and are now electing to replace missing teeth with bone-anchored implant-supported prostheses. The implant fixture or bone-anchored unit and the transmucosal element intimately unite biochemically as well as mechanically to healthy living tissue. The entire entity, along with the dental restoration, has been referred to as a Tissue-Integrated Prosthesis (T.I.P.).

Due to the better than 95% success rate reported by Brånemark and colleagues[5] and the approximately 38 million edentulous people in the United States alone, the percentage of patients seeking to improve their dental health and ultimately the quality of their lives is increasing dramatically. As the median age of the population increases along with life expectancy, the number of problem denture patients will certainly rise. Long-term denture patients suffer severe loss of the residual alveolar ridge bone and consequently they lose denture retention.

It is the authors' viewpoint that restoring partially and fully edentulous patients with advanced ridge reduction presents the most complex and technically demanding procedures in dentistry today.

Experience has shown that the team approach is a highly effective, practical method of providing patients with a successful Tissue-Integrated Prosthesis. The osseointegration team consists of a skilled surgeon, a prosthodontist or restorative dentist, the dental technician, and specially trained dental assistants and hygienists. The technician must be a knowledgeable and informed part of this team, for not only are they responsible for diagnostic setups, guidestents, and the eventual fabrication of the final prosthesis, but they are often called upon as consultants for the development of the initial treatment plan. In providing these services, the authors have experienced great satisfaction in being an important part of this team. As the use of osseointegration implants increases, the skilled implant technician will be asked to provide technical support to meet the challenging demands of the profession and the patients they help serve.

Since the early 1980's we have seen the implant prosthesis progress from being a novelty to an integral part of laboratory procedures. At the time of this publication, four implant systems were chosen to illustrate restoration design and fabrication concepts. These systems were selected based on their general widespread use; together they provide most of the materials and components needed to restore normal function and esthetics. These four systems are: Brånemark System; Core-Vent; Interpore IMZ; and Integral. In addition, several "after market" companies also provide compatible components offering alternative design features. The skilled technician can use this book as a reference for most dental implant systems as the authors have seen a definite similarity between all of them. They each contain impression copings, implant replicas for use in the master cast, and prosthetic components used in the final prosthesis. The handling procedures for the components are very similar in nature and can be mastered relatively quickly.

Experience has been a great teacher. Having successfully completed thousands of implant restorations, the authors feel that sharing the experience and knowledge they have gained will prove of great help to the dental technician and clinician as well. Working closely with many leading prosthodontists in the development of prostheses design and concepts has been an exciting, rewarding, and enriching experience. We now want to share this knowledge with our colleagues and to all who continue to participate as active members of the health care team. It is the authors intention that this book supply practical answers for today's problems and open many new doors for the future.

References

1. Brånemark P-I, Zarb GA, Albrecktsson T, eds. *Tissue-Integrated Prostheses: Osseointegration in Clinical Dentistry*. Chicago, Ill: Quintessence Publishing Company; 1985;1:11.

2. Balshi T. Osseointegration for the periodontally compromised patient. *Int J Pros*. 1988;1:51-58.

3. Sullivan D. Prosthetic considerations for the utilization of osseointegrated fixtures in the partially edentulous arch. *Int J Oral Maxillofac Imp*. 1968;1:39-45.

4. Jemt T. Modified single and short span restorations supported by osseointegrated fixtures in the partially edentulous jaw. *J Pros Dent*. 1986;55:243-248.

5. Adell R. Long-term treatment results. In: Brånemark P-I, Zarb GA, Albrecktsson T, eds. *Tissue-Integrated Prostheses: Osseointegration in Clinical Dentistry*. Chicago, Ill: Quintessence Publishing Company; 1985:175-186

Chapter 2

Surgical Guidestents

After a patient is accepted for implant treatment, it is recommended that a surgical guidestent be fabricated.[1] A guidestent is a device that is used during the first stage surgery to aid the surgeon in properly positioning and angulating the guide drill. When a guidestent is used as fabricated, the fixtures can be placed ideally .to insure optimum esthetics for the tissue-integrated prosthesis.[2]

During the pretreatment planning, the oral surgeon and restorative dentist use all available information; this may include CAT scans, lateral view cephalometrics, pan-radiographs, and diagnostic casts. The number of fixtures and the correct diameter and length[3] can be determined from this information.

Although the guidestent show the ideal placement of the fixture, the availability and quality of bone may dictate otherwise.

In this chapter, six different laboratory-fabricated guidestents are selected for their variety of use and design. From the authors experience, a successful esthetic restoration has its start when a surgical guidestent is utilized.

Partially Edentulous Mandibular Anterior Guidestent

This tooth-supported stent with plastic sleeves offers good cross-arch stability, ideal fixture placement and angulation. Figure 2-1 is a diagnostic cast showing ideal position for six implants.

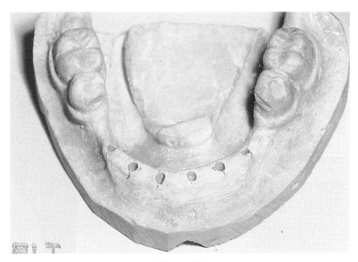

Fig. 2-1

Holes are drilled to simulate ideal fixture angulation. Dowel pins and plastic sleeves (Whaledent International) are placed on the lubricated cast. It is important that the plastic sleeves do not extend below the tissue level. The plastic fin at the middle of the sleeve must be incorporated in the stent material. Tooth undercuts are then blocked out on the cast with wax.

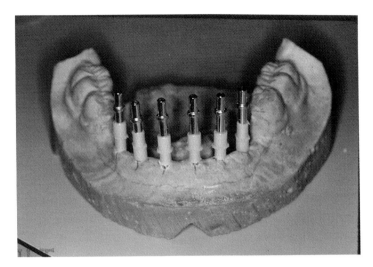

Fig. 2-2

Ivory-colored Triad (Dentsply International) material is adapted to a six millimeter height around plastic sleeves and to the occlusal surface of posterior teeth. It is then light cured in the Triad curing unit, removed from the cast, finished and polished.

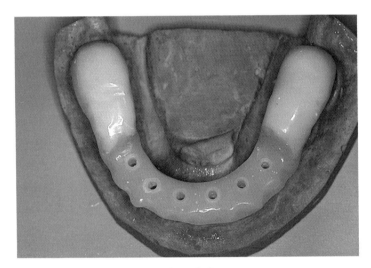

Fig. 2-3

This finished guidestent with the pins replaced illustrates ideal fixture placement and angulation.

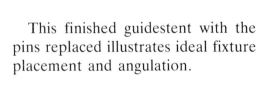

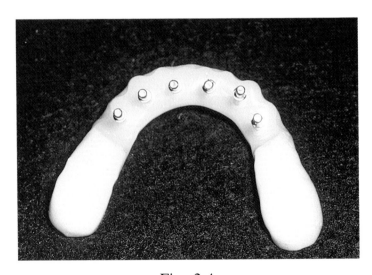

Fig. 2-4

Partially Edentulous Mandibular Posterior Guidestent

This study cast has markings for two implant sites. Using a #8 bur, the holes are drilled with a lingual inclination of the long axis of the drill bit.

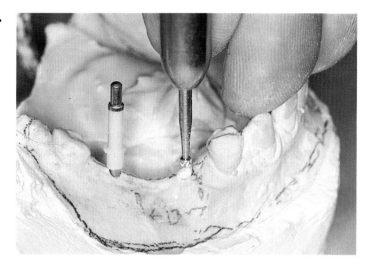

Fig. 2-5

The holes are cleaned, the cast is lubricated and tooth undercuts are blocked out.

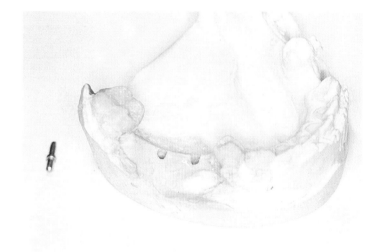

Fig. 2-6

Dowel pins and sleeves are placed on the prepared cast.

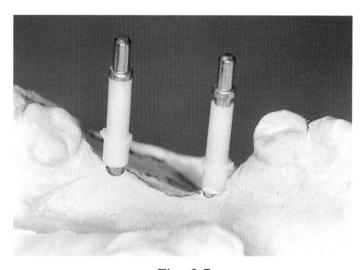

Fig. 2-7

The best possible angulation was determined by setting denture teeth in proper alignment, and with pins perpendicular to the ridge. Denture teeth are drilled, shaped to fit, covered with Triad Gel (Dentsply International) and light cured.

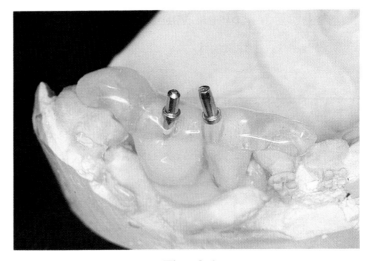

Fig. 2-8

The two-fixture guidestent after final finish and polish.

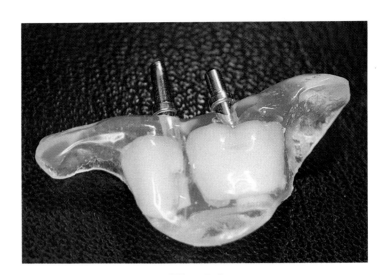

Fig. 2-9

Fully Edentulous Mandibular Guidestent with Maximum Opening Apparatus

It was determined before surgery that this patient had extreme difficulty in keeping her mouth open to accommodate the surgical procedure.

This shows a cast with six fixture positions marked with the required lingual and labial border of the guidestent.

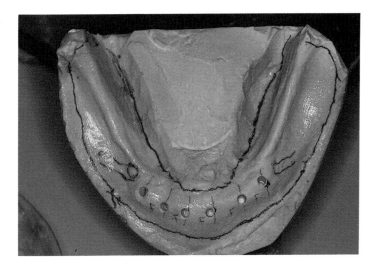

Fig. 2-10

Holes are drilled with five millimeter spacing and checked with a millimeter gauge. Dowel pins and sleeves are placed on the lubricated cast.

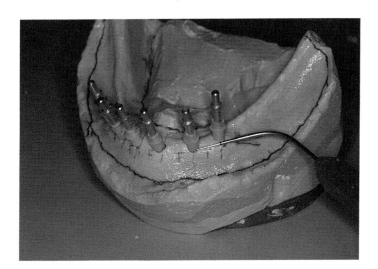

Fig. 2-11

Pink Triad material is adapted around sleeves and edentulous areas.

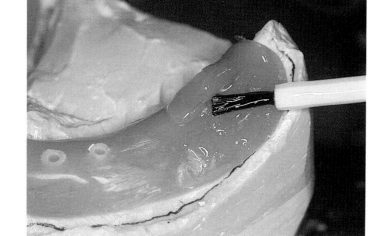

Fig. 2-12

The stent is removed from the cast after curing, then finished and polished.

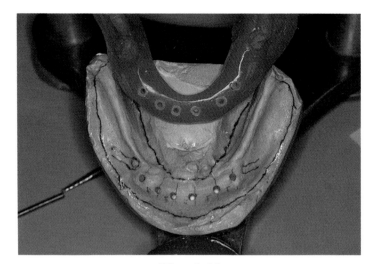

Fig. 2-13

The maxillary cast with Triad baseplate is articulated with the prepared mandibular guidestent cast using a prescribed pin setting.

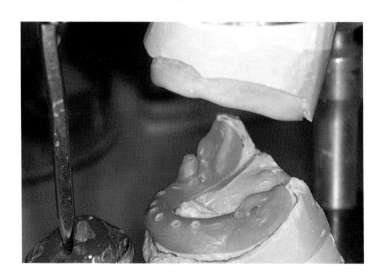

Fig. 2-14

Triad material is added to posterior areas of the baseplate and guidestent and then light cured.

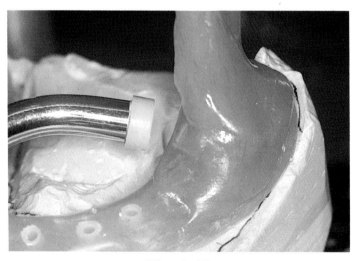

Fig. 2-15

The final connection is then completed and cured.

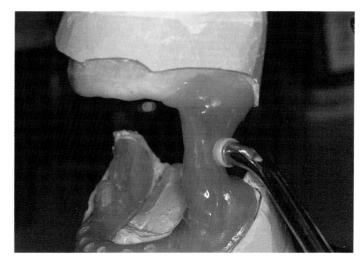

Fig. 2-16

The custom guidestent is removed, cleaned, and ready for delivery.

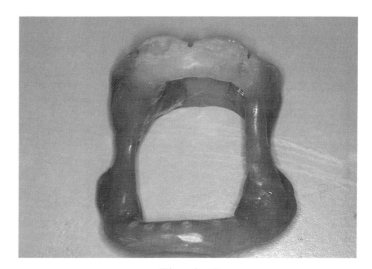

Fig. 2-17

The tissue side of the stent is inspected before insertion.

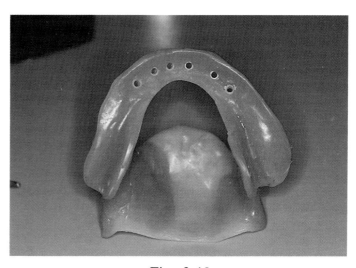

Fig. 2-18

Tea Cup Duplicate Denture

Many times, a restorative dentist will prescribe a duplicate of the patient's denture to be used as a surgical guidestent. This guidestent dictates the maximum facial position for the fixtures, while allowing the surgeon lateral and lingual freedom of placement and angulation. The authors have found the following technique to be quick and less expensive than fabricating a new denture.

The basic materials needed include: large cup which has been lubricated, alginate impression material, spatula, bowl, and the patient's denture.

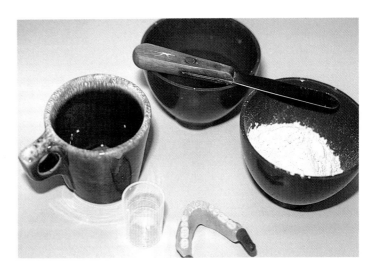

Fig. 2-19

The denture has wide wax extensions added to both distal heels.

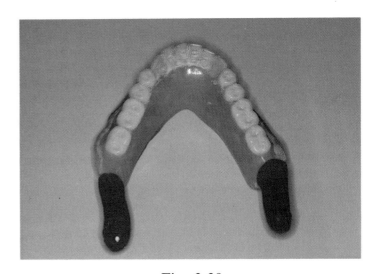

Fig. 2-20

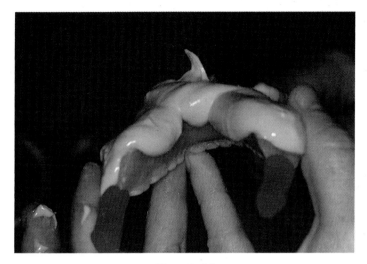

Alginate is mixed and carefully adapted to capture the fine details of the denture.

Fig. 2-21

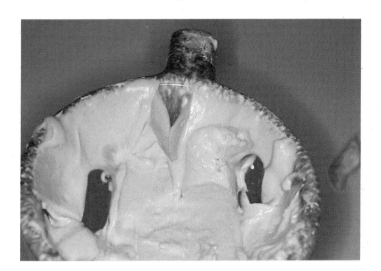

The denture is submerged in the cup of wet alginate until only the wax extensions are visible.

Fig. 2-22

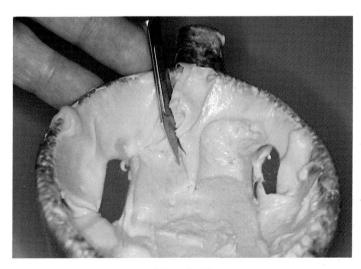

When the alginate is set, it is indexed for accurate replacement.

Fig. 2-23

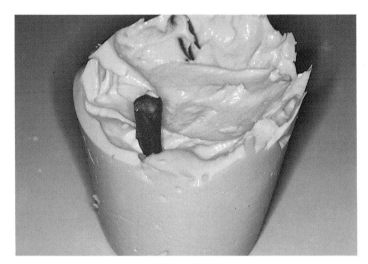

The entire impression is removed from the cup.

Fig. 2-24

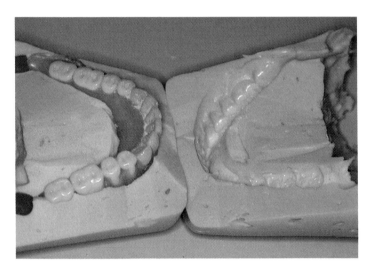

Using a razor knife, the alginate is carefully cut in half down to the denture.

Fig. 2-25

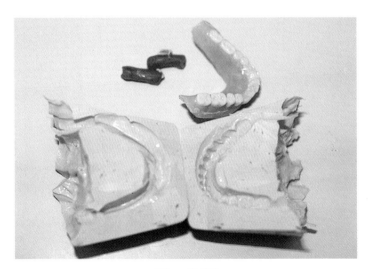

The denture with wax extensions is removed and the impression is inspected for accuracy.

Fig. 2-26

The two halves are reassembled and placed back in the cup, using the index.

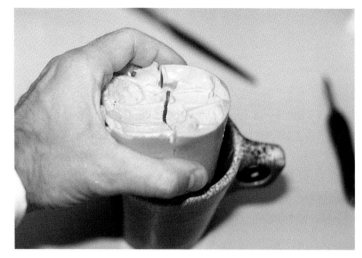

Fig. 2-27

Clear orthodontic resin (L.D. Caulk) is mixed according to recommended powder and liquid ratios.

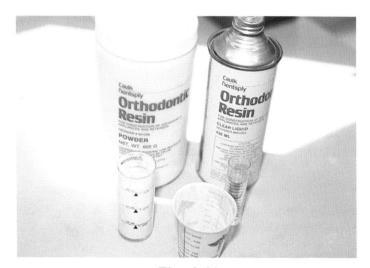

Fig. 2-28

Resin is poured down one side of the impression until it rises up through the other opening.

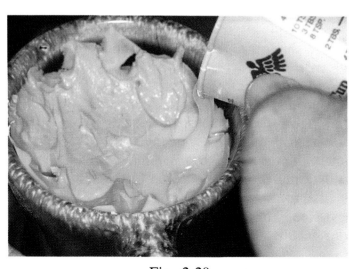

Fig. 2-29

A vibrator is used to increase the flow of the material and reduce air bubbles.

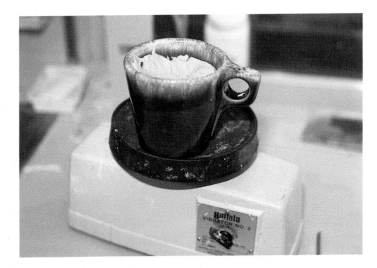

Fig. 2-30

This shows the newly processed, unfinished, clear duplicate denture.

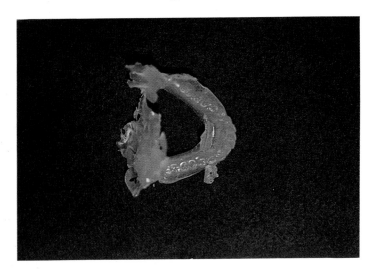

Fig. 2-31

The duplicate denture is finished to correct border length and hollowed from the left second bicuspid around the anterior section to the right second bicuspid, leaving the buccal/labial aspect of the teeth intact. The section that is removed is determined by the position of the mental foramina. An 18 gauge stainless steel wire is added to the anterior section for strength.

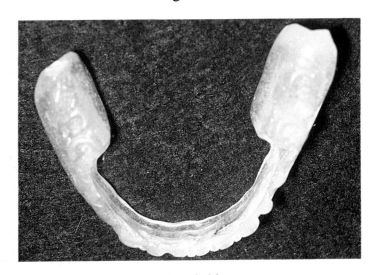

Fig. 2-32

Spare Denture Stent

A set of spare dentures is modified by removing the palatal and lingual acrylic as indicated. A labial wire is added to each arch for increased strength, and the denture stents are finished and polished. These stents provide an esthetic guide while offering the same functions as the clear duplicate denture.

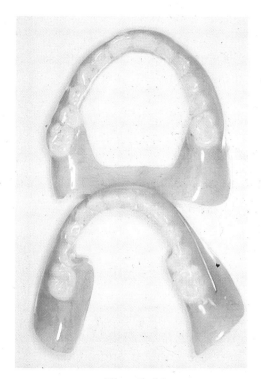

Fig. 2-33

Radiographic Splint

The primary function of the radiographic splint is to provide presurgical diagnostic information. In this application, a metal ball bearing was used. The measurement of the actual ball is compared to the ball size in the radiograph. The size difference between the two balls is used to create a ratio which is equivalent to the distortion factor in the radiograph.[4] In a cephalometric radiograph, it is helpful in determining fixture placement and angulation.

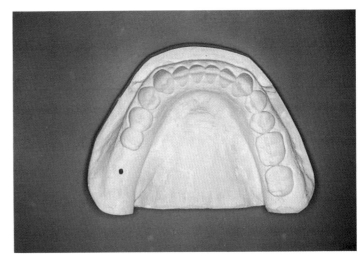

This is a mandibular cast with marking for one implant site.

Fig. 2-34

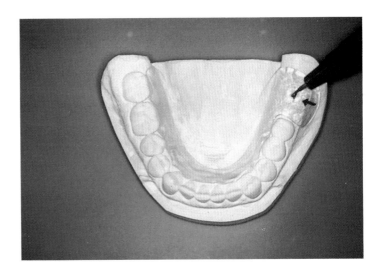

The acrylic splint is fabricated with a saddle over the implant area. The implant site is marked on the splint.

Fig. 2-35

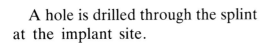

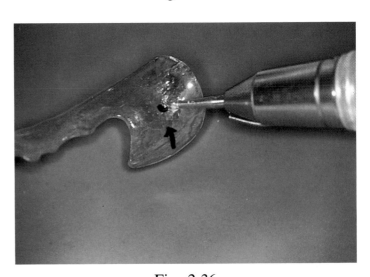

A hole is drilled through the splint at the implant site.

Fig. 2-36

The splint is placed back on the cast and the metal ball bearing is attached to the implant site with self-curing acrylic.

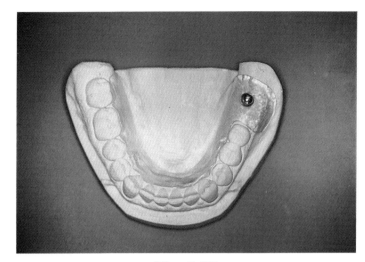

Fig. 2-37

This slows the finished splint with the radiographic ball bearing.

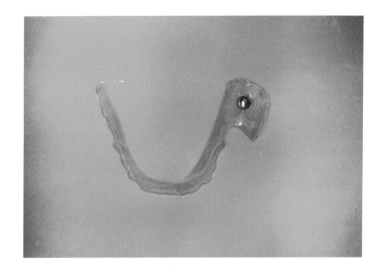

Fig. 2-38

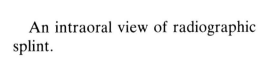An intraoral view of radiographic splint.

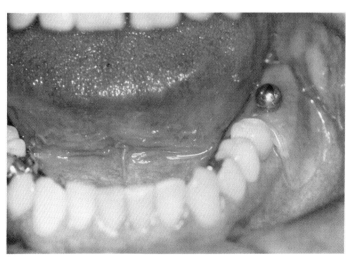

Fig. 2-39

Here the radiographic splint is shown on a panradiograph.

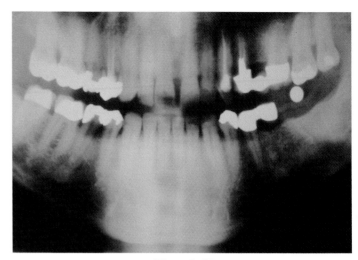

Fig. 2-40

References

1. Edge MJ. Surgical placement guide for use with osseointegrated implants. *J Pros Dent.* 1987;57:719-722.

2. Blustein R, Jackson R, Rotskoff K, Coy RE, Godar D. Use of splint material and the placement of implants. *Int J Oral Maxillofac Imp.* 1986;1:49-47.

3. Engelman MJ, Sorensen JA, Moy P. Optimum placement of osseointegrated implants. *J Prosthet Dent.* 1988;59:467-473.

4. Hobo S, Ichida E, Garcia L. *Osseointegration and Occlusal Rehabilitation.* Chicago: Quintessence Publishing Company; 1990:65-73.

Chapter 3

Full Mandibular Reconstruction Using The Brånemark System

The first application for the implant-supported prosthesis or tissue-integrated prosthesis (TIP) was the fully edentulous mandible. This has become known as the traditional Brånemark System fixed removable bridge.

Clinical implant studies conducted by Brånemark et al.[1] and Adell et al.[2] have indicated the effectiveness and long-term success of this restoration. The first edentulous patient was successfully treated in 1965 by closely following the established osseointegration principles.[3] The patient showed excellent dentate function, as well as soft and hard tissue conditions after a 15-year follow-up was completed. A 25-year follow-up study indicated equally encouraging results. By combining extensive documentation of biological research analysis with their equally thorough proven methods of prosthodontic reconstruction, the Swedish researchers have truly given the world an invaluable resource.

The authors' modification of the original Toronto design by Zarb et al.[4] has produced over 550 bridges with only three fractures. These failures have been attributed to inadequate thickness of the metal surrounding the terminal abutment cylinder in conjunction with severe bruxism and/or extremely strong masticatory forces.

As stated earlier, the need for proper treatment planning cannot be emphasized enough. Radiographs, study casts, and any information available should be used to construct a surgical guidestent for the placement of the fixtures.

There are several types of prosthetic teeth that have been successfully used in the denture bridge format. These include Ivoclar (Ivoclar); Bioblend, Bioform (Dentsply); Myerson (Nobelpharma); and Vita (Vita Zahnfabrik).

The results can be outstanding if care is taken in the selection of shade and mold.

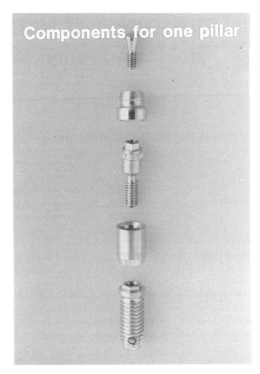

The hardware for the Branemark System includes the titanium implant fixture, the titanium abutment and abutment screw. The prosthetic components at the top are the gold cylinder and gold screw. The Brånemark System prosthetic gold cylinder has a melting temperature of 2350° F. The alloy selected for the frame must have a melting temperature well below this figure.

Fig. 3-1

This is a cross-sectional view of the assembled hardware without the gold cylinder.

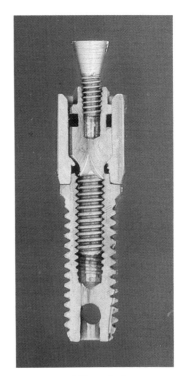

Fig. 3-2

The metal of choice is widely accepted to be a Class IV gold alloy. A successful lower-cost metal is a palladium-based alloy with Class IV properties.

The authors strongly recommend a heat-cured acrylic for use in the final denture bridge prosthesis. Good results have been obtained by the high impact Lucitone 199 (Dentsply).

In cases of restricted vertical dimensions where mechanical retention is limited, it is necessary to use a metal treatment to attain retention. Such treatments include: Lee Metal Primer (Lee Pharmaceutical); the Silicoater (Kulzer); and 4-Meta (Parkel).

The rest of the chapter will show in detail the fabrication procedures of the traditional denture bridge from the impression to final insertion.

Following second stage surgery, the correct abutments are placed.

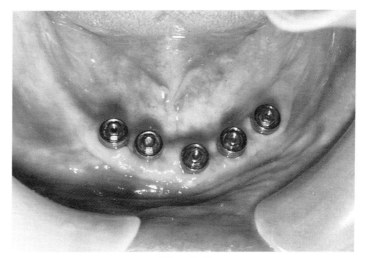

Fig. 3-3

The clinician takes a full arch impression of the fixture abutments and all edentulous areas. Soft tissue anatomical landmarks should be reproduced for diagnostic evaluation. The preliminary cast is fabricated from the impression.

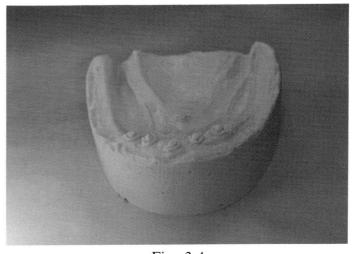

Fig. 3-4

Square impression copings are positioned on each fixture site and secured with sticky wax. This will indicate the proper height and width necessary for the window portion of the custom tray.

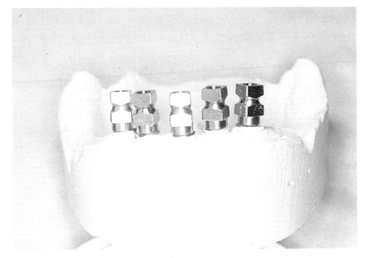

Fig. 3-5

Impression copings are blocked out with utility wax facilitating an easy removal from the custom tray.

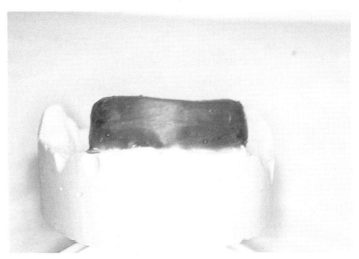

Fig. 3-6

A heavy body acrylic tray is heated and vacuum formed over the entire cast. The tray is separated from the cast and finished to proper dimensions. An access window is cut into the top of the coping block out until all screws have clearance.

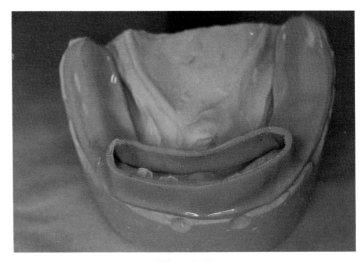

Fig. 3-7

Impression copings are screwed into place with guidepins; a light wrap of dental floss or similar material is adapted to all copings intraorally. The coping/floss bridge is luted together with small amounts of DuraLay until the entire pattern is complete. This technique stabilizes the copings within the impression, increasing the accuracy of the pickup.

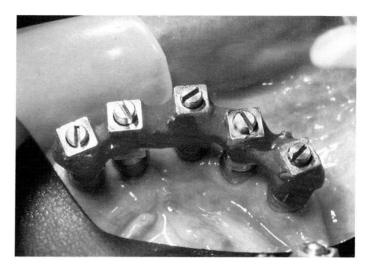

Fig. 3-8

The tray is tried in the mouth to determine the fit over the copings and DuraLay bridge. Impression material is loaded into a syringe and a custom tray. The fixture area is adapted first, using the syringe, then the impression is taken following normal protocol. Screw access holes should be identified and exposed. The guidepins are unscrewed and the impression removed and inspected. All coping surfaces engaging the fixture must be cleaned. Impression material covering any metal margin indicates inaccurate component contact and the impression should be retaken.

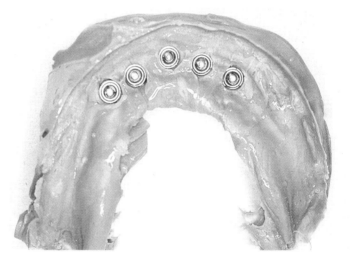

Fig. 3-9

After the impression is deemed accurate, guidepins are used to secure brass replicas into place.

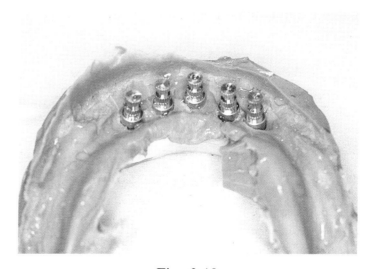

Fig. 3-10

Impressions are poured in improved die stone and occlusal rims are fabricated. The mandibular rim is implant-supported using at least two cut down impression copings (a square impression coping as shown on patient's right is cut in half as shown at left). This is done routinely, since the vertical height of the coping is usually taller than the occlusal plane to be registered.

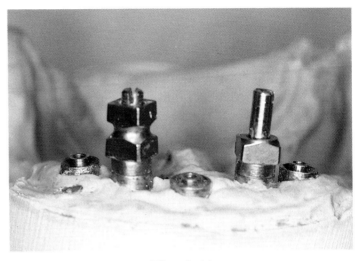

Fig. 3-11

Copings are blocked out with wax from the tissue up to the underside of the square portion of this cylinder-like component. All subsequent brass replicas are covered with wax up to the height of the coping block-out. The cast is then lubricated. Triad light-cured material or cold cure acrylic is adapted around the square copings. Any area distal to the last replica is given tissue contact up to the retromolar pad; giving better support in those areas not stabilized by the impression coping. After curing, finish and lightly polish with pumice. Wax is then luted to the base at the recommended heights (18 mm anteriorly and half way up the retromolar pad posteriorly).

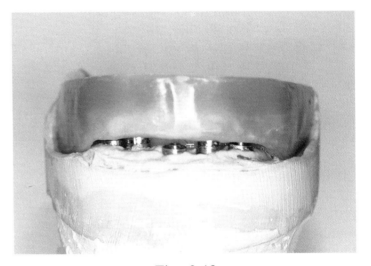

Fig. 3-12

Gold screws, or guide pins that have been cut down below the occlusal height, can be used to secure this intraorally.

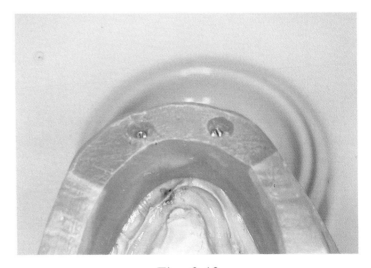

Fig. 3-13

The fully edentulous casts are mounted on a semi-adjustable articulator using the occlusal rims.

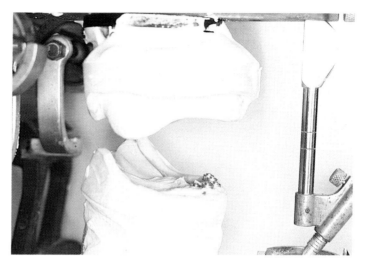

Fig. 3-14

Using the information from the occlusal rims, denture teeth (Bioblend, Dentsply) are set and verified intraorally. A verification jig is fabricated to check the accuracy of the impression. Gold cylinders are mounted and secured with guide pins. The cylinders are blocked out up to the concavity, and at least 6 mm of DuraLay is built on top of this. After the DuraLay has cured, the jig is checked for passive fit on the model. When this has been satisfied, the verification jig is tried intraorally. There must be a perfect passive fit of each cylinder to each abutment. If the jig is inaccurate, the offending cylinder must be located and sectioned. It is then re-DuraLayed in the mouth. At this time, the altered cast technique must be performed (see Figures 3-44 and 3-45).

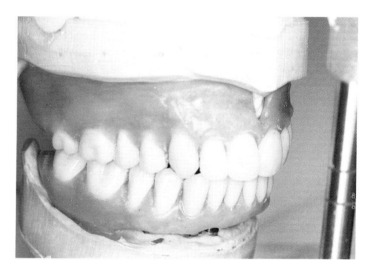

Fig. 3-15

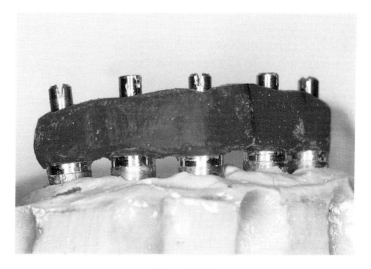

Fig. 3-16

The authors strongly recommend setting all fully edentulous restorations in a full-balanced occlusion. This will prevent premature wear of teeth, but, more importantly, will prevent the "popping off" of teeth which usually occurs in the maxillary if this is not done. This important step can save hours of future chair time.

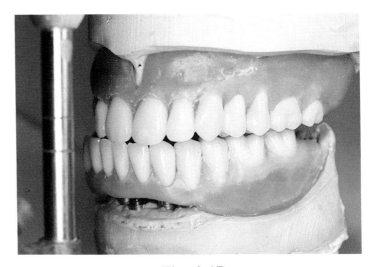

Fig. 3-17

Figure 3-17 shows the balancing side with all the lingual cusps of the upper in contact with the buccal cusps of the lower. Incisal edges of the upper and lower are also in contact.

When fit, function and esthetics are verified, the lower cast is keyed in preparation to receive a matrix.

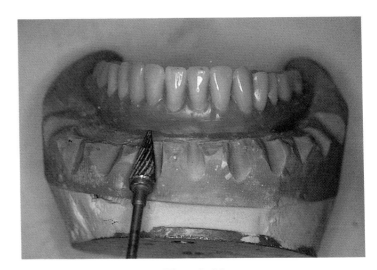

Fig. 3-18

The cast is lubricated and the plaster matrix is formed. Plaster is placed around the buccal and labial of the wax-up, engaging the keys on the cast and the occlusal surface of the posterior and incisal edges of anterior teeth.

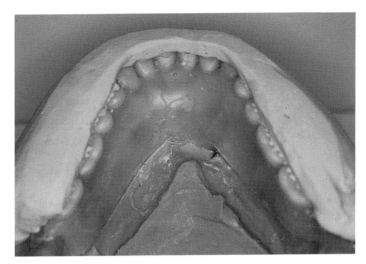

Fig. 3-19

After the plaster has set, wax is boiled away and the light-cured base is removed. The matrix with teeth in place is returned to the keyed cast. The frame is now ready to be built within this master cast, matrix, and tooth configuration. Red lines on the cast indicate a 15 mm cantilever. Since the second molars go beyond this mark, they will be omitted.

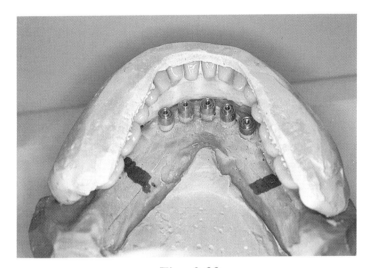

Fig. 3-20

The gold cylinders are placed on the brass replicas and secured with guide pins. Red utility wax is used to block out the bottom portion of cylinder up to the point where the cylinder has its concavity. There is also a slight block out of the ridge of the cast distal to last cylinder. Blue rope wax is then used to outline the red block out wax. This will act as a trough to contain the wet DuraLay and prevent it from spilling onto the cast.

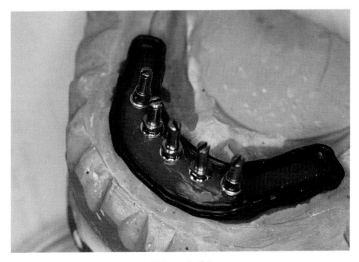

Fig. 3-21

This is a lingual view of screw-retained cylinders with trough and block-out.

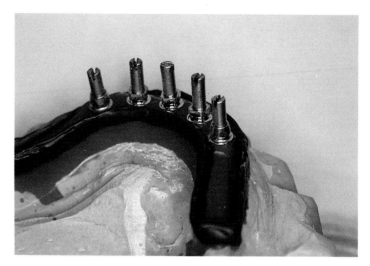

Fig. 3-22

Using the brush method, the trough is filled with DuraLay. Screws can be lightly coated with petroleum jelly to aid in easy removal.

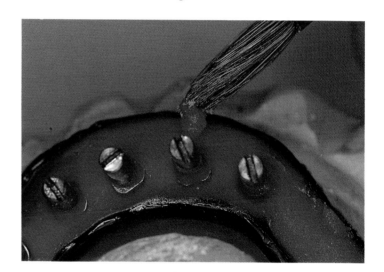

Fig. 3-23

When the DuraLay has set, all wax is steamed off. The overbuilt frame is now ready for contour.

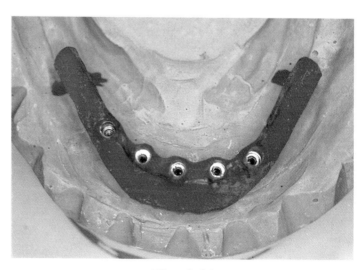

Fig. 3-24

Using a variety of burs, the Dura-Lay frame is shaped and smoothed. A lingual wall of at least 4 mm and bucco-lingual width of 3 mm is essential for strength. Since the terminal cylinders bilaterally are extreme stress points, it is recommended that 5-6 mm in height be built circumferentially in this immediate area.

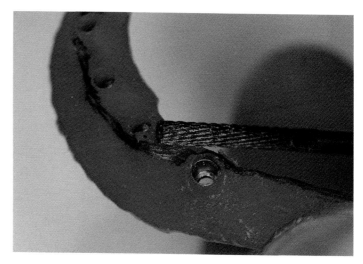

Fig. 3-25

The plaster matrix is fitted to the master cast. The relationship of teeth to frame is checked for proper support. The transition from frame to teeth should be as smooth as possible to eliminate any discrepancies or irregularities that might irritate the tongue.

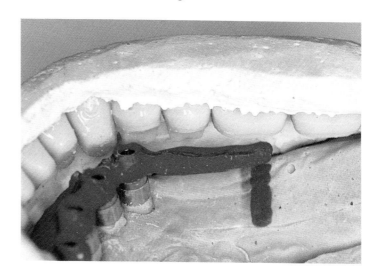

Fig. 3-26

Because of the uncontrollable stresses of large or even small amounts of DuraLay, it is necessary to cut every section between each cylinder. This will allow each cylinder to sit perfectly on each brass replica.

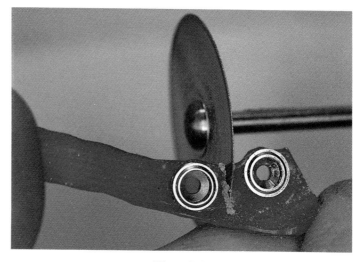

Fig. 3-27

Exploded view of sectioned frame.

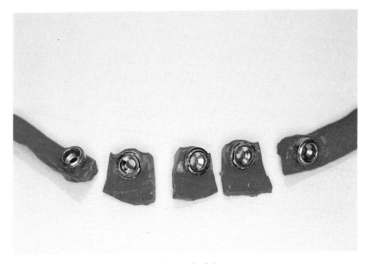

Fig. 3-28

Each section is waxed to fill any voids, and a finish line is incorporated. Careful attention should be given to the cylinders. No wax or debris should be in or around the gold component from the double ring configuration to at least .5 mm up on the outer circumference.

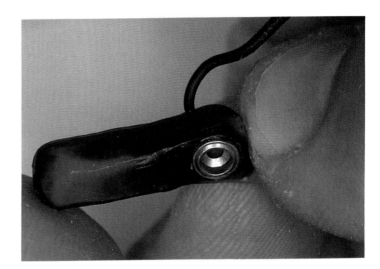

Fig. 3-29

A nylon bristle brush is used as a final check for clearing any wax or DuraLay from the inner portion of the cylinder.

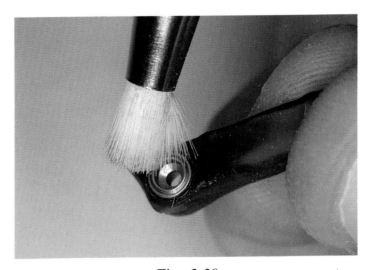

Fig. 3-30

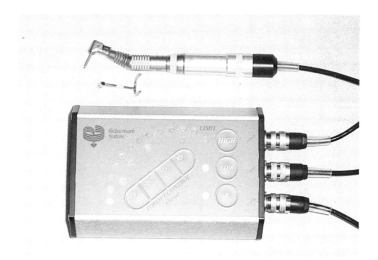

To insure equal tightening force, the Nobelpharma electronic torque driver is used for all subsequent steps. This guarantees that all cylinders are tightened to 10 N cm.

Fig. 3-31

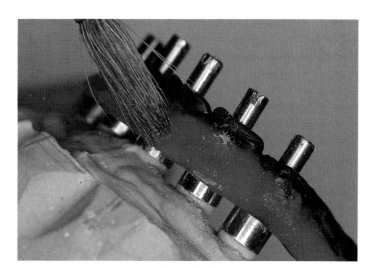

Each wax and DuraLay section is secured to the master cast with guide pins in their proper positions. Small increments of DuraLay are then used to lute the sections together.

Fig. 3-32

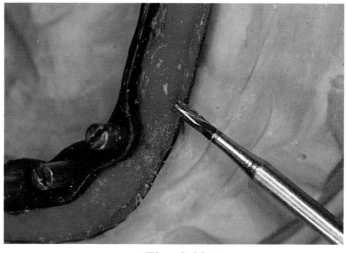

After the resin has set, a carbide bar is used to cut a bezel finish line around the buccal and lingual of the frame. This will act as a retentive device to grab the processed acrylic and eliminate any separating of the acrylic at the metal-acrylic junction. It is recommended that the resin frame set overnight to relieve all stresses and insure a proper fit.

Fig. 3-33

Loops are added to the frame for acrylic retention. Eighteen gauge rope wax is wrapped around a straight-shanked instrument, then slid off. Each ring which touches the frame should be luted with sticky wax. This not only retains the acrylic, but adds overall strength to the frame.

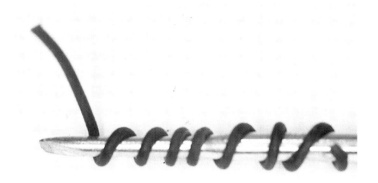

Fig. 3-34

The matrix is fitted to the master cast, and any teeth that contact the loops of the frame must be reduced.

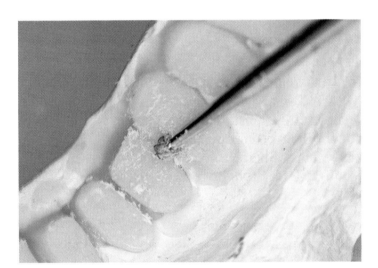

Fig. 3-35

This is the buccal view of the finished wax-up. Beads (Veneer Lock, Taub Products Co.) have been added to further increase the acrylic retention.

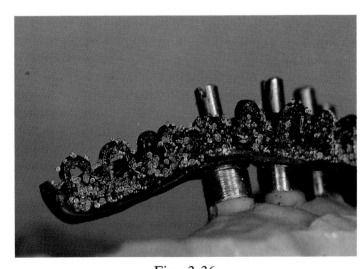

Fig. 3-36

This is the lingual view showing the smooth finish for ease in casting and polishing.

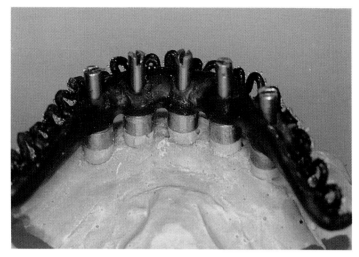

Fig. 3-37

Twelve gauge sprue wax is luted to the tip of the lingual walls between each cylinder. A wax bar is connected to the terminal end of each cantilever, with two extra sprues added vertically.

NOTE: Sprue wax should not be placed directly behind gold cylinders.

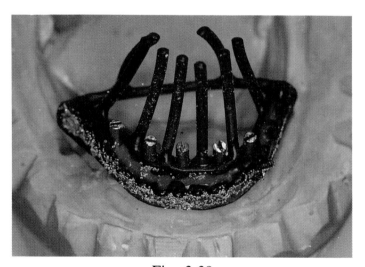

Fig. 3-38

The DuraLay frame is invested following manufacturer directions (Beauty Cast, Whip Mix Co.). Care should be taken that the investment comes from the underside and pushes its way through the top. This will insure against air being trapped in the cylinder.

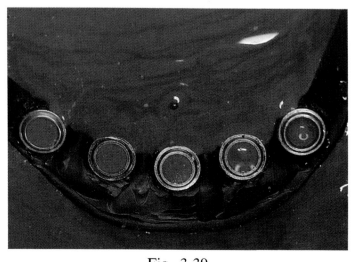

Fig. 3-39

The ring should be bench set for one hour. It is then placed in a cold burn-out oven and burned out at 500° F for one hour. The temperature is then raised to 1150° F, held for 30 minutes, and the ring is then cast in a type IV gold alloy (T-IV-L, Nobelpharma). After bench cooling, the ring is carefully broken out and the casting is cleaned. DO NOT sand blast the gold cylinders.

This shows the cast gold framework with sprues cut off. The bar at the distal of the cantilevers is left attached until final processing of the restoration is complete. This will help to prevent warpage during lab procedures, especially during packing and breakout.

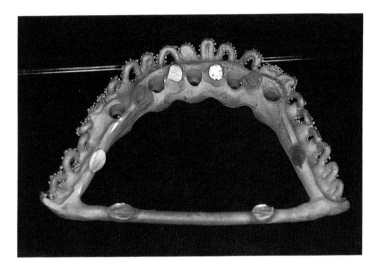

Fig. 3-40

The underside of the frame must be highly polished and as smooth as possible. This will prevent plaque and other debris from collecting in these areas.

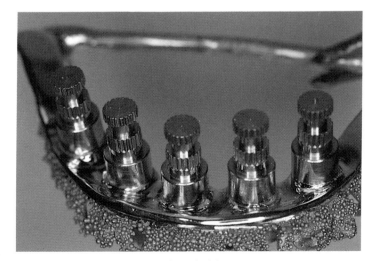

Fig. 3-41

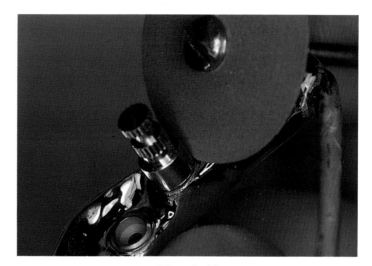

Fig. 3-42

When finishing and polishing the underside of the frame, brass replicas or a protective cap should be used to avoid marring or nicking the metal interface surface of the gold cylinder.

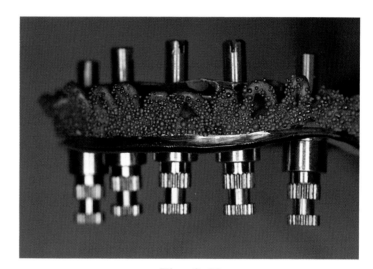

Fig. 3-43

This shows the highly polished finished gold frame.

Even though the frame fit the master cast, it proved inaccurate when brought to the mouth. It is sectioned at the offending site and DuraLayed in the mouth for the correct position.

NOTE: If a verification jig had been used, these soldering steps would not have been necessary. The jig would have pointed out the impression inaccuracy and a new impression could have been taken before the laboratory procedures were started.

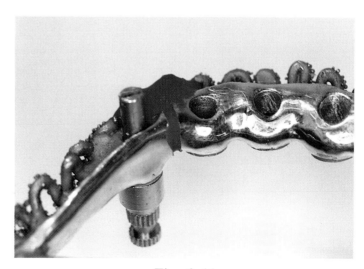

Fig. 3-44

Since the frame was sectioned and DuraLayed, it will now not fit the master cast. Locate the offending area and carefully remove the brass replica from the cast; connect a new one to the frame by a guide pin. When the frame is placed on the cast, the new replica must sit passively in the bored-out area. There should be no stone touching any part of the new replica. When the frame will seat in this fashion, it is secured by all guide pins and stone is used to secure the new replica. This will produce the new altered master cast. The frame can now be soldered.

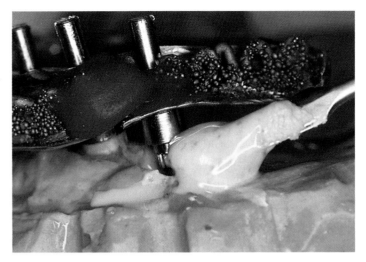

Fig. 3-45

Using the plaster matrix as a guide, the denture teeth are waxed to the gold frame. Occlusion and esthetics are checked, and it is recommended that a final intraoral check be done.

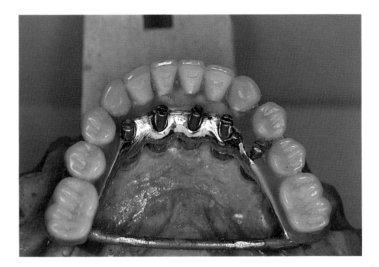

Fig. 3-46

After final verification, brass replicas are attached to the frame using guide pins.

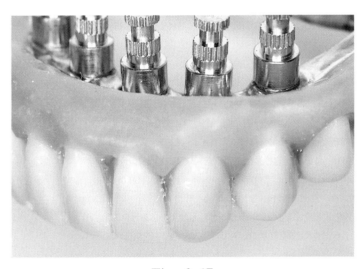

Fig. 3-47

A small plaster model is fabricated. This will aid greatly in the breakout procedure.

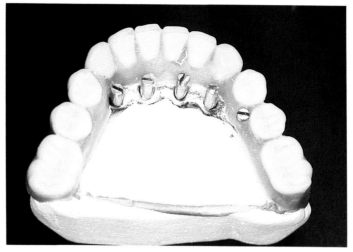

Fig. 3-48

The restoration is now half-flasked in the usual manner. It may be necessary to relieve protruding guide pins with wax or a silicone-type material so that they will not bind and prevent the flask halves from separating.

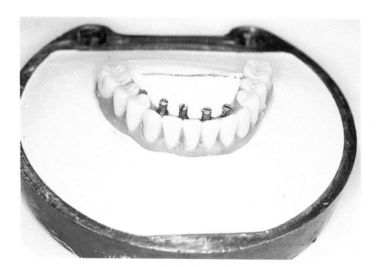

Fig. 3-49

The second half of the flask is prepared in the conventional manner.

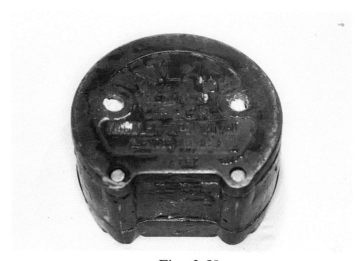

Fig. 3-50

The flask is placed in boiling water and all wax is eliminated. Extra retentive cuts can be made in the denture teeth. Paint both sides of the flask with a separating medium (Al-Cote, Densply).

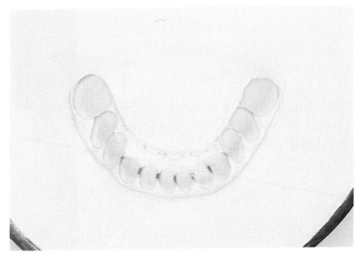

Fig. 3-51

This is the opposite side of the flask, showing the gold framework.

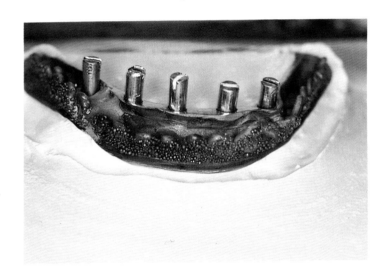

Fig. 3-52

The Silicoater (Kulzer) is used for increased acrylic-to-metal bond.

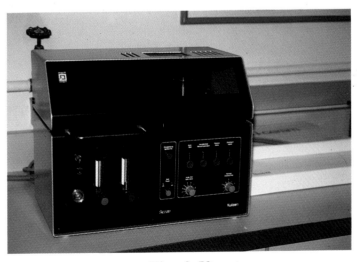

Fig. 3-53

Since the gold frame has a tendency to show through the pink acrylic, it is necessary to opaque the metal.

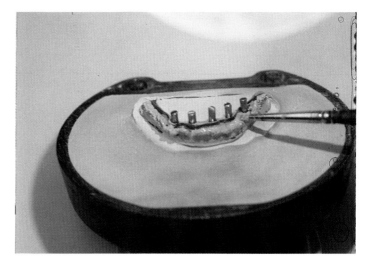

Fig. 3-54

Tooth-colored acrylic (Jet, Lang Dental Mfg.) is mixed, applied to the screw access holes, and the flask is closed. This prevents pink acrylic from appearing on the occlusal surfaces of the teeth. The flask is immediately opened and any flash material is trimmed away.

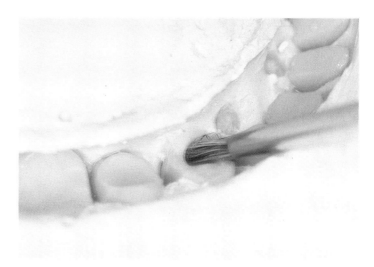

Fig. 3-55

Lucitone 199 acrylic (Dentsply) is formed into a roll and placed on both sides of the flask. Separating cellophane is placed between the two halves and the entire flask is closed and pressed at 3500 PSI. The flask is opened, the cellophane is removed, and all flash acrylic is removed. New cellophane is applied and the flask is pressed again. This procedure is continued until all flash material is eliminated.

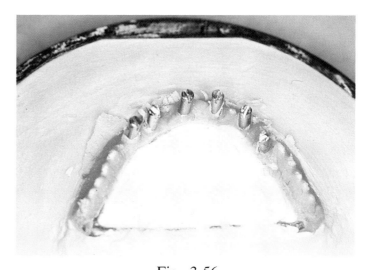

Fig. 3-56

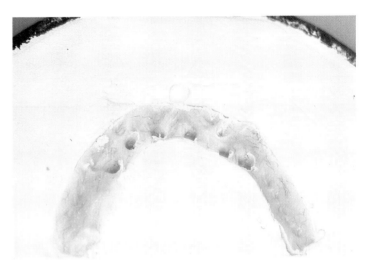

Before final closure, remove the cellophane and apply a light coat of monomer to the acrylic surfaces, close the flask, press, and cure at 165° F for nine hours.

Fig. 3-57

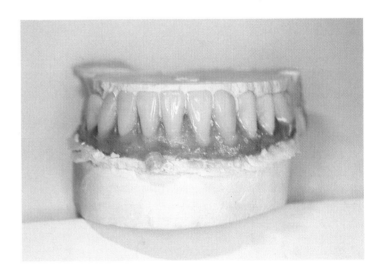

After the curing cycle is complete, the flask is separated, and the processing model with prosthesis is carefully removed.

Fig. 3-58

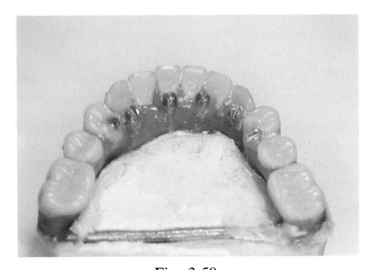

A lingual view of the processed TIP.

Fig. 3-59

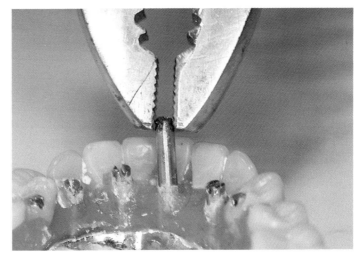

It is sometimes necessary to use pliers in removing guide pins from the processed acrylic.

Fig. 3-60

An alternate method of removing guide pins is to use a punch on the threaded end of the guide pin. This punch could be fabricated from a standard laboratory steel-shanked bur. A concavity is formed on one end using a #8 bur.

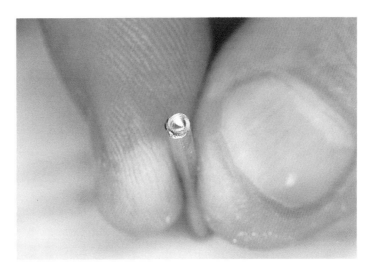

Fig. 3-61

The concavity holds the punch on the screw, preventing the bur from sliding and marring the gold cylinder.

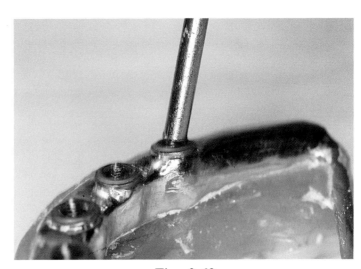

Fig. 3-62

The distal stabilizing bar is removed.

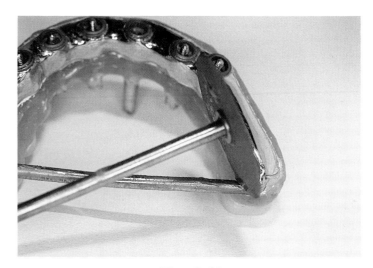

Fig. 3-63

The processed upper and TIP lower are remounted on the articulator and processing errors are removed. It is important to recheck the balanced occlusion at this time.

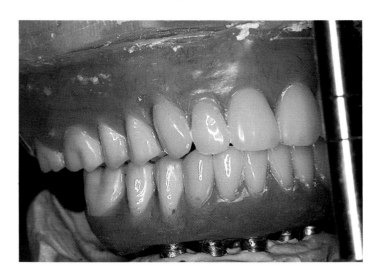

Fig. 3-64

The upper and lower are finished, polished, and ready for insertion.

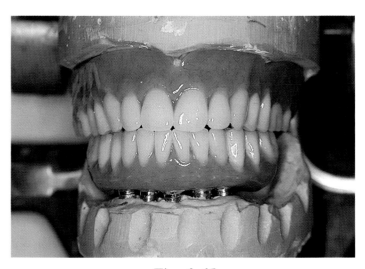

Fig. 3-65

This intraoral view of the TIP shows good framework fit, hygiene access areas, and esthetics.

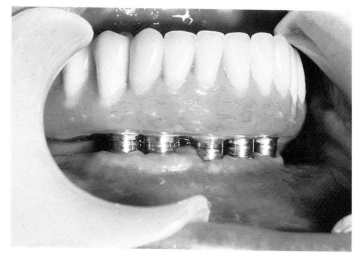

Fig. 3-66

Prosthodontic rehabilitation is complete.

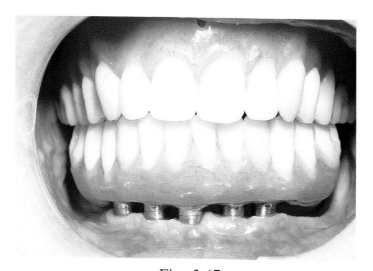

Fig. 3-67

References

1. Brånemark PI, et al. Osseointegrated implants in the treatment of the edentulous jaw—experience from a ten-year period (Monograph). Stockholm: Almqvist and Wiksell; 1977.

2. Adel R, et al. A 15-year study of osseointegrated implants in the treatment of the edentulous jaw. *Int J Oral Surg*. 1981;6:387.

3. Brånemark P-I. Introduction to Osseointegration. In: *Tissue-Integrated Prosthesis*. Chicago: Quintessence Publishing Company. 1985:47.

4. Zarb GA, Jansson T. In: Brånemark P-I, Zarb GA, Albrektsson T, eds. *Tissue-Integrated Prostheses: Osseointegration in Clinical Dentistry*. Chicago: Quintessence Publishing Company; 1985:311-315.

Suggested Reading

Zarb G, Jansson T. Laboratory procedures and protocol. In: Brånemark P-I, Zarb GA, Albrektsson T, eds. *A Tissue-Integrated Prostheses: Osseointegration in Clinical Dentistry*. Chicago: Quintessence Publishing Company; 1985: Chapter 17.

Chapter 4

An Overview of the Porcelain-To-Metal Technique

The critical factors in the use of porcelain are: meticulous fabrication and laboratory maintenance of a precision framework. It is imperative that correct procedures be followed continuously through to completion of the prosthesis. The design of the substructure should incorporate accurate anatomical dimensions with strong, rigid connectors.[1] In a full-arch framework, a palatal bar is included in an effort to prevent warpage. Thin areas of metal are avoided in all ceramo-metal frames. This minimizes flexure and metal fatigue, both leading to potential porcelain fracture. As discussed in Chapter 3, the Brånemark System gold cylinder has a melting temperature of 2350° F, and any metal selected for use must be well below this temperature. The castable components in the Core-Vent and IMZ systems permit the use of base, noble, or high noble alloys.

Ideally, the porcelain veneer should be 2 to 2.5 mm thick in order to insure a high compressive strength. With proper framework design, facilitating optimum porcelain veneer coverage, the restoration has a high degree of rigidity.[2] This allows even distribution of occlusal loading forces to the osseointegrated fixtures.

With the exception of areas of weak trabecular bone,[3] there are no significant studies which prove that the lack of shock-absorbing qualities inherent in porcelain should contraindicate its use as a treatment modality. In the event that a porcelain restoration is ultimately required when there is trabecular bone, a period of controlled loading should be prescribed, using an acrylic resin prosthesis.[4] Bone remineralization has been observed occurring up to one year after fixture placement in the mandible, and up to 18 months in the maxilla.[5] Bone remodeling continues for many years. Using an acrylic provisional provides a damping effect which allows additional dense lamellar bone to form. This gives the fixture an increased resistance to overloading, increasing the probability of a successful ceramic bridge.

Minimal resorption of the alveolus in partially edentulous mandibles, and the restrictive space limitations present in the anterior of the maxilla, often requires a ceramo-metal restoration. The use of custom shade matching and oral hygiene maintenance, along with the qualities of resisting staining and occlusal wear, are potential favorable characteristics of a porcelain restoration.

Fully Edentulous Maxillary Tissue Integrated Prosthesis Using Porcelain-Fused-To-Metal

This master impression contains seven impression copings. Before attaching the brass replicas with guide pins, each coping is closely inspected for debris present on the surface.

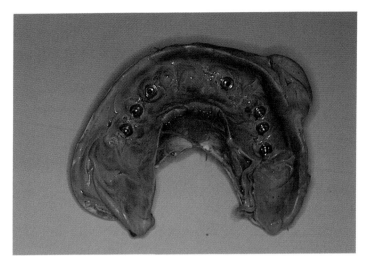

Fig. 4-1

The master cast is poured with improved die stone. A full arch impression should be extended to duplicate good ridge morphology and anatomic landmarks.

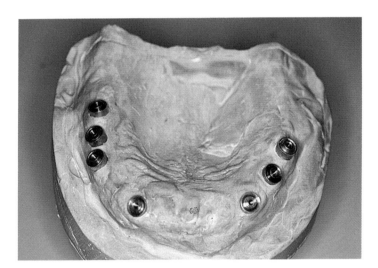

Fig. 4-2

The maxillary and mandibular casts are articulated.

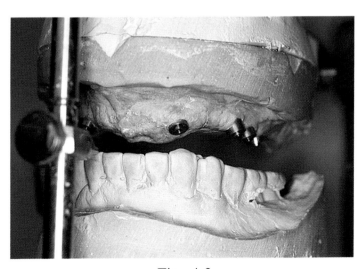

Fig. 4-3

A clear acetate vacuum-formed matrix taken from a model of the patient's temporary restoration is fitted to the articulated upper cast using the palette as a guide.

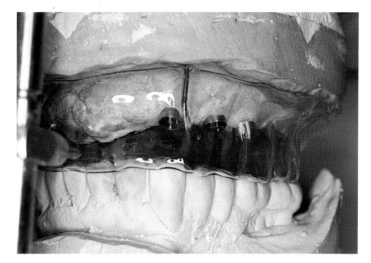

Fig. 4-4

DuraLay resin is used to connect the gold cylinders on the lubricated maxillary cast.

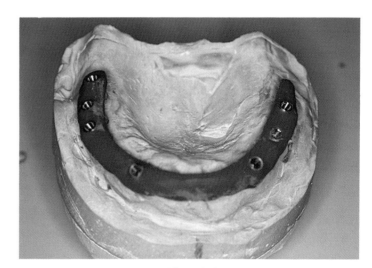

Fig. 4-5

When the acrylic has the desired thickness of 4 mm, the clear matrix is used to establish buccal, labial and lingual borders. Excess acrylic is trimmed until the matrix will seat easily on the model.

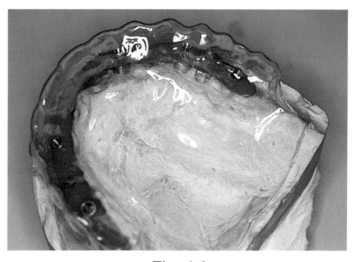

Fig. 4-6

The acrylic is cut into four sections, and each section is waxed to final contour using the clear matrix as an anatomic guide. After all wax has been added, the pieces are joined together with fresh resin and allowed to bench set for one hour. A palatal bar is added with a #8 gauge sprue attaching the distal molars. This bar will help the frame resist distortion from the heat and stress of the porcelain oven.

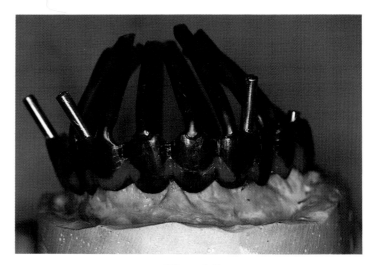

Fig. 4-7

After careful investing with a high heat investment (Ceramigold, Whip Mix Co.), the ring is allowed to bench set for one hour, it is then placed in a cold burn-out oven and the temperature raised to 500° F and held for one hour. The oven is reset for 1450° F and again held for one hour. The pattern is cast in a high noble alloy (WY, Williams Co.) and allowed to bench cool. The metal frame is then cleaned and finished. During metal finishing, it is very important that brass replicas or similar components be fastened to the cylinders with guide pins. This preserves the integrity of the cylinders and encourages a fine finish line at the junction of the frame and cylinders. This procedure is repeated for any additional metal work and also for the final polishing of the frame.

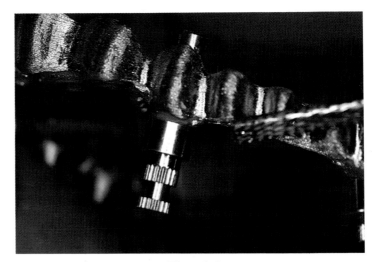

Fig. 4-8

At the metal try-in stage, the frame does not fit passively on all fixtures.[6] The metal is sectioned through the left central and the palatal bar, both pieces are reseated with gold screws, and a DuraLay index is made for soldering. A solder model with brass replicas is made from the indexed frame. Using the frame as an index, the inaccurate brass replicas are removed from the master cast. New brass replicas are fastened to the frame with guide pins and refitted to the master cast, making sure that no stone is in contact with the brass replicas. The frame is secured with guide pins and stone is poured around the new replicas. This completes the altered cast technique. The case is then removed from the new master cast, invested with high heat solder investment, and soldered (see Chapter 10). The metal is then cleaned, finished, and returned for a second metal try-in.

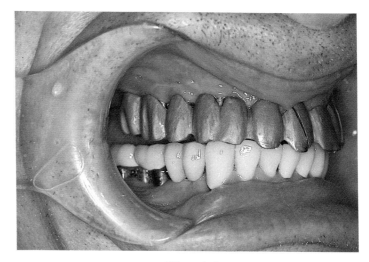

Fig. 4-9

A lateral view cephalometric radiograph verifies the intimate and passive fit that is required from the frame.

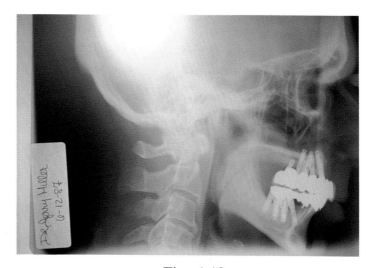

Fig. 4-10

After the frame has been degassed and the custom opaque applications are complete, the gingival and incisal porcelains are built up. Full cervical contour is evident, along with slightly lengthened incisal edges. The porcelain must be contoured and condensed accurately on the first bake. Multiple firings of full arch porcelain prosthesis increase the chance of frame distortion.

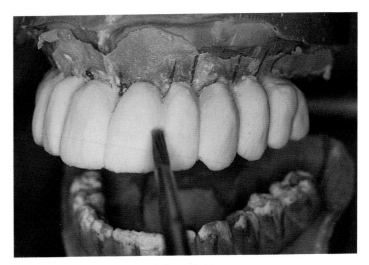

Fig. 4-11

The guide pins used during the porcelain buildups maintain the cleanliness of the screw and cylinder interface. After baking, the ceramic particles are very difficult to remove from the inside portion of the cylinder.

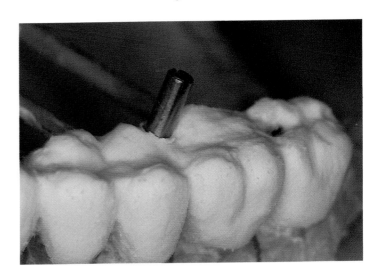

Fig. 4-12

A bisque bake trial is completed, with some adjustments being made to equilibrate the occlusion.

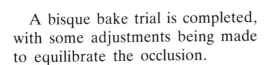

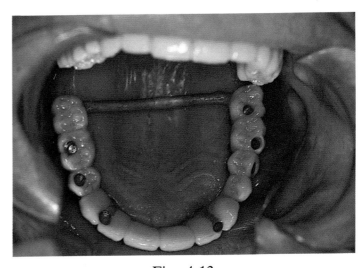

Fig. 4-13

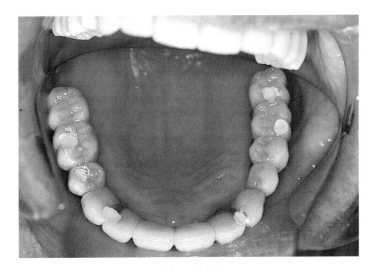

The porcelain is then glazed and the metal is polished. The palatal bar is cut off at this time and the prosthesis is screwed into place, with the access holes temporarily sealed with cotton pellets and cavitt.

Fig. 4-14

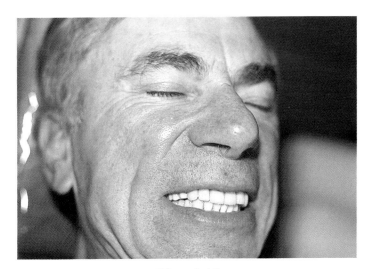

Prosthodontic rehabilitation is now complete, with full muscle support evident in the cheek and lip area.

Fig. 4-15

Lip retractors reveal good soft tissue adaptation and all screw access holes cosmetically hidden from view.

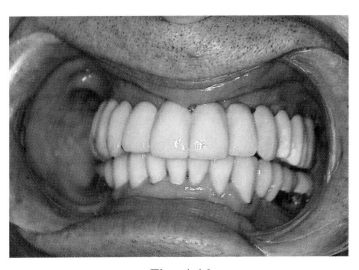

Fig. 4-16

Posterior Quadrant Reconstruction
With a Natural Tooth Abutment
And the IMZ Implant

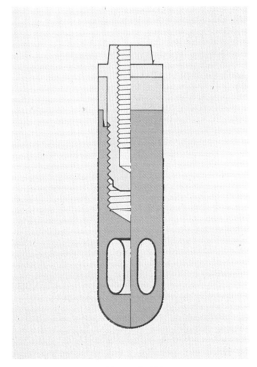

This cross-sectional schematic diagram illustrates the internal relationship of the implant components.

Fig. 4-17

Components include from left: titanium screw and intramobile element for 4.0 mm diameter fixture; titanium screw and intramobile element for 3.3 mm diameter implant; 4.0 mm impression post; 2.0 mm impression post with model replica; impression post and model replica for 3.3 mm diameter implant.

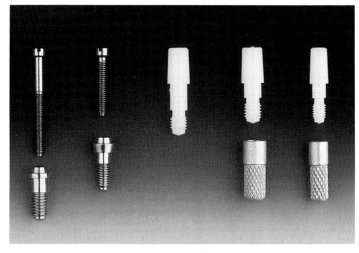

Fig. 4-18

From left: 4.0 mm implant cylinder; second phase healing screw; titanium healing screw; placement head; titanium transmucosal extension; and intramobile element (IME).

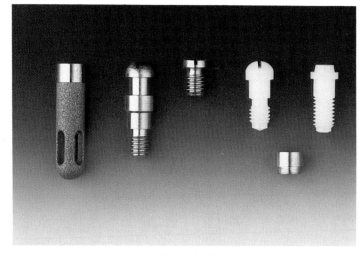

Fig. 4-19

This shows the implant uncovered and ready for placement of transmucosal extension and intramobile element.

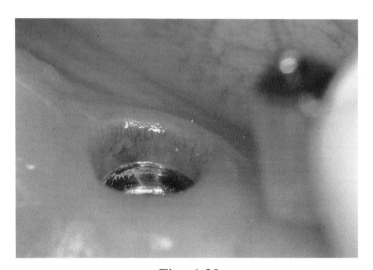

Fig. 4-20

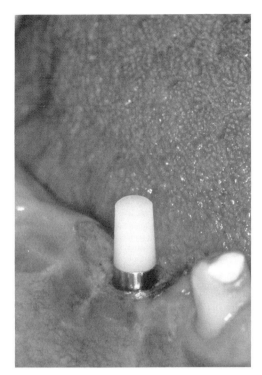

The impression post is shown screwed into place.

Fig. 4-21

A full arch view of the master impression with model replica attached.

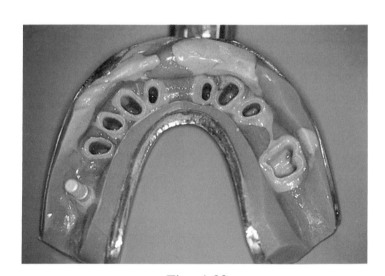

Fig. 4-22

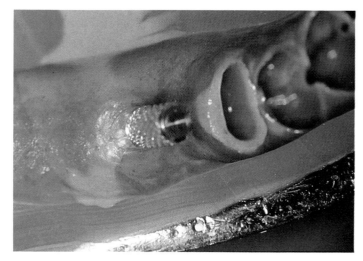

Fig. 4-23

The distal view illustrates the impression post with the model replica properly placed back into position.

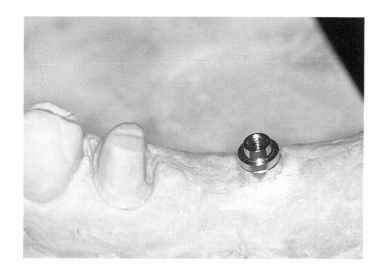

Fig. 4-24

The master cast is poured and the laboratory IME is screwed into the fixture replica.

The maxillary and mandibular casts are articulated.

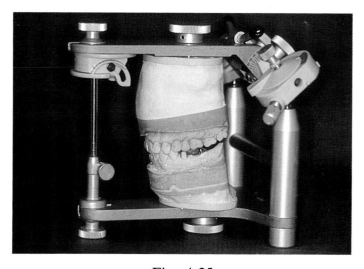

Fig. 4-25

The occlusal height dictated by the master casts is used to correctly adjust the length of the titanium screw, the plastic waxing sleeve, and the tube and screw attachment.

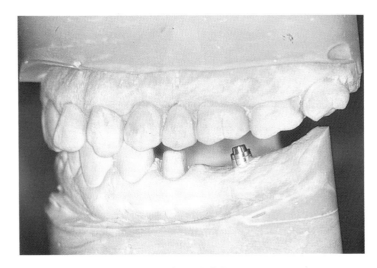

Fig. 4-26

The height of the waxing sleeve is reduced by removing the desired length from the middle of the sleeve. This technique maintains the preformed ends which fit the neck of the screw and the head of the IME. The two halves are then reattached with DuraLay resin and the component design is completed.

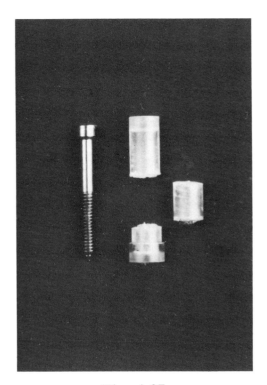

Fig. 4-27

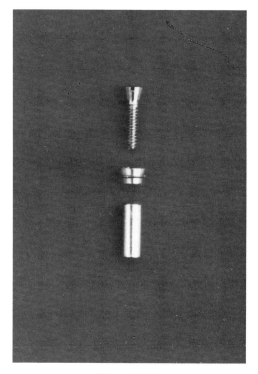

Fig. 4-28

The tube and screw attachment (Cendres and Metaux, Sterngold) incorporates a ferrule which has a precision fit with the head of the screw and the rim of the tube. The integrity of these components is essential to the success of the bridge.

The attachment is placed at the distal of the bicuspid abutment. It should be parallel to the path of insertion of the implant screw. The coping is waxed with the attachment enveloped in a cast position. The wax pattern is designed with an extracoronal block which has walls with a five degree taper. A surveying table or similar device is used to check the degree of taper on the three outside walls, ensuring the fit and draw of the overcasting.

The pattern is fitted with a special casting screw to maintain the threads of the female tube. It is then sprued up and invested in a high heat phosphate investment. The casting ring is burned out, cast in a noble alloy (Naturelle, Jeneric/Pentron) and allowed to bench cool.

The casting is carefully devested and fitted to the bicuspid die. The extracoronal block is then polished. The secondary component containing the plastic waxing sleeve and screw is now fabricated.

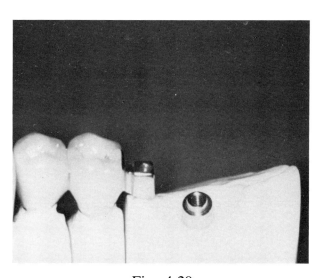

Fig. 4-29

The extracoronal block is coated with lubricant and the ferrule is put to place with the screw. A resin shell is formed around the ferrule and the entire extracoronal block. Using resin, the balance of the connection is finished between the waxing sleeve and the resin-coated block. Final contours are waxed, the pattern is sprued up, invested, and cast in a noble alloy. The casting is devested and fitted precisely to the implant replica and extracoronal block. The two-piece assembly is now ready.

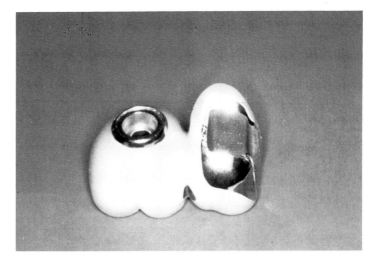

Fig. 4-30

The schematic diagram illustrates all components and crown contours in correct harmony. Note the fixing screw adjusted slightly out of occlusion. The tip of the screw reaches the recommended depth inside the IME.

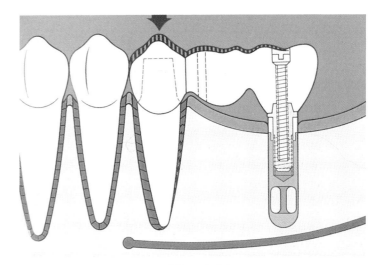

Fig. 4-31

The metal frame is degassed, and opaque is applied in two stages. The gingival and incisal porcelains are now blended, with particular care being taken to keep the screw holes clean and free of porcelain. Note the shape and contour of all finish lines.

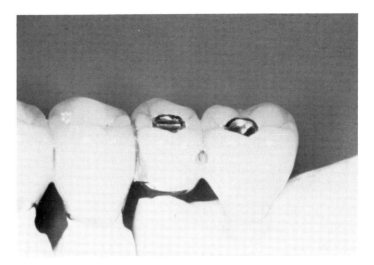

Fig. 4-32

All porcelain work is completed. The three-unit bridge is tried in and the occlusion is adjusted.

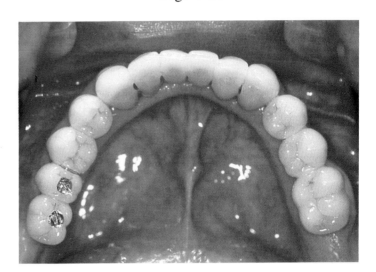

Fig. 4-33

After a final glaze and polish, the bridge assembly is complete.

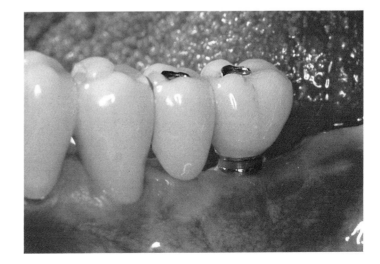

Fig. 4-34

Partially Edentulous
Reconstruction Using
The Core-Vent System

A quadrant impression shows Core-Vent implant replicas (CV BH3) seated firmly on the impression posts (CV BC3). A small amount of sticky wax is used to insure the replica does not move.

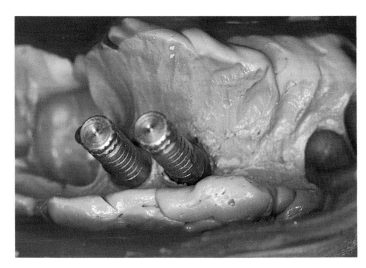

Fig. 4-35

The impression is boxed with wax and ready for a stone pour.

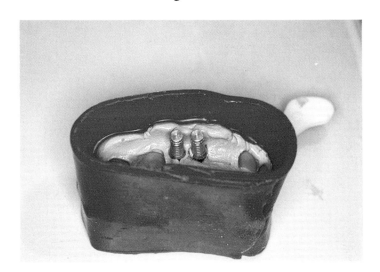

Fig. 4-36

The master cast is separated, cleaned and trimmed.

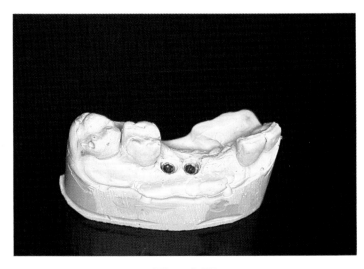

Fig. 4-37

A close-up view of the implant replicas reveals a clean metal surface and accurate reproduction of soft tissue surrounding the fixtures.

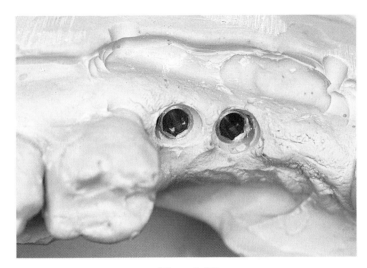

Fig. 4-38

This view shows the Core-Vent impression posts (CV #BC3) on the left, with castable post on the right (CV #PC3).

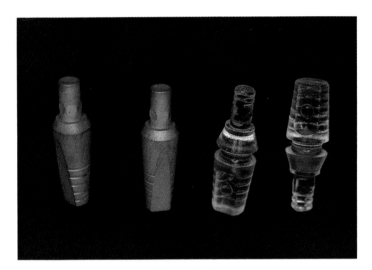

Fig. 4-39

The PC3 patterns are seated in the implant replicas. The articulated casts show the buccal inclination present. The PC3 will be modified lingually to enhance the esthetics of the implant-supported bridge.

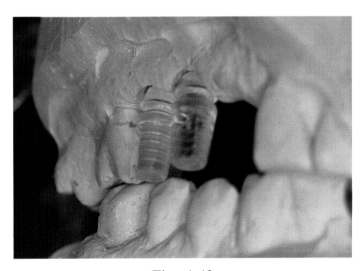

Fig. 4-40

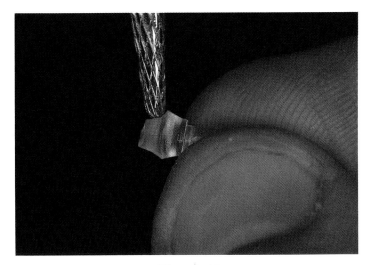

Fig. 4-41

A carbide bur is used to reduce the size of the two PC3 patterns to the desired shape.

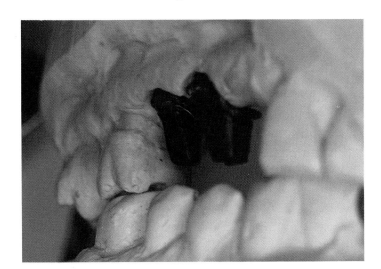

Fig. 4-42

Crown and bridge wax is added to the shortened PC3 patterns to form a parallel path of insertion for the bridge. Adequate occlusal space should be maintained to allow ideal ceramo-metal contours to be restored.[7]

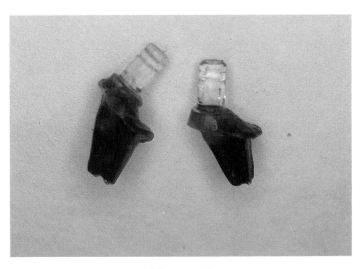

Fig. 4-43

The posts are removed from the model and the final touch-up contours are completed in wax. The two patterns are sprued up invested in a high heat phosphous investment (Ceramigold II, Whip Mix Corp). After correct burn-out procedures, the ring is cast using SFC metal (Jeneric-Pentron Corp.), following the manufacturer's directions.

The castings are carefully devested, with special attention being paid not to violate the integrity of the post portion of the pattern. The tissue side of the post is highly polished and the coronal aspect is finished with a diamond bur.

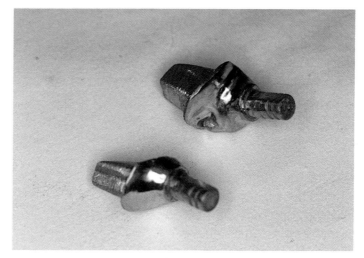

Fig. 4-44

The posts are shown seated on the master cast. Note the finish line prepared just above the tissue level. This promotes a good emergence profile as well as a very esthetic bridge. The two modified PC3 posts are ready for cementation.

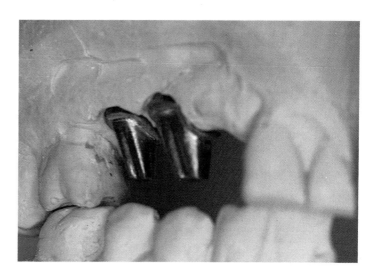

Fig. 4-45

An impression is taken of the cemented posts and a master cast is poured and pindexed. The entire area of the bridge is contained in one large die to preserve the accuracy needed for a well-fitting overcasting.

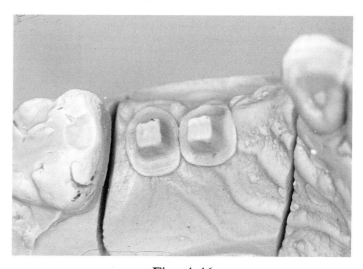

Fig. 4-46

The stone posts are treated with die hardener (Rock Set, Jelenko Co.). The wax pattern substructure is created on each post, initially. This enables the technician to control the marginal fit and coping contour to a fine degree. The pontic, with a small holding tab, is then placed, and all the units are connected with wax. The sprues are attached, and investing and casting procedures are completed as in Figure 4-9.

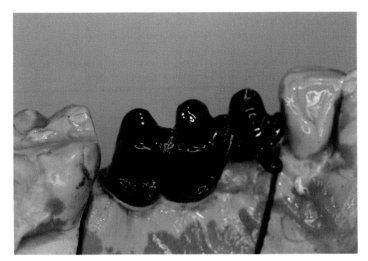

Fig. 4-47

The casting is carefully devested and inspected for defects.

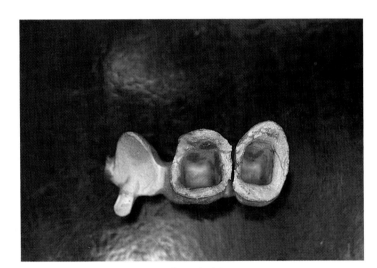

Fig. 4-48

Metal finishing procedures are completed and checked on the model. The interproximal area here is extremely narrow and must be kept open to promote good hygiene.

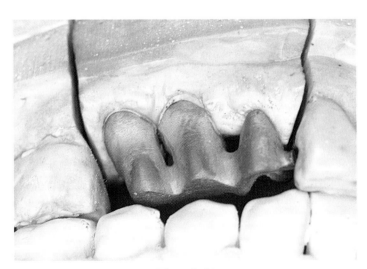

Fig. 4-49

The casting is sandblasted, degassed, and a first wash of opaque is applied.

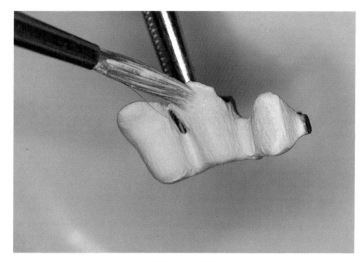

Fig. 4-50

A second layer of opaque enhances the coloration and masking properties.

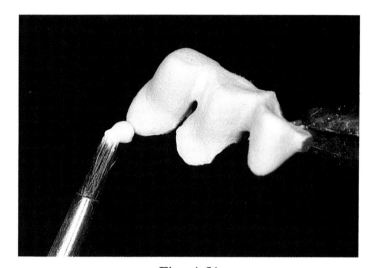

Fig. 4-51

A small piece of wet tissue paper is adapted to the cuspid pontic area. This step helps to create good gingival contour upon removal. The opaqued frame is seated on the cast and the porcelain buildup is started.

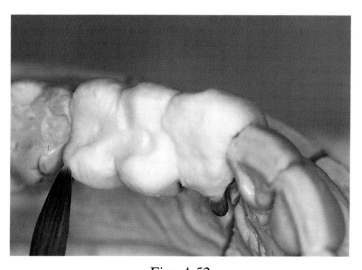

Fig. 4-52

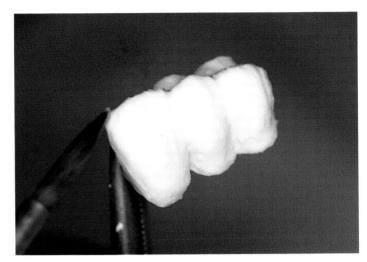

The final crown contours are completed. The bridge is now ready for the porcelain baking cycle.

Fig. 4-53

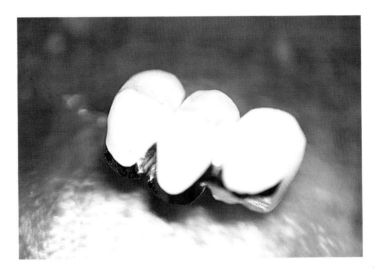

This lingual view of the bridge shows the porcelain finished and glazed. The metal is sand-blasted internally and highly polished on the crown surface.

Fig. 4-54

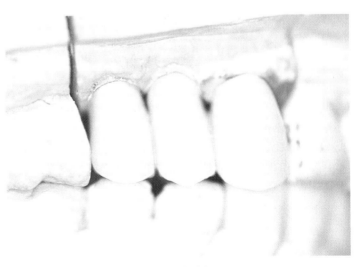

When a buccal view is taken, the bridge shows excellent marginal fit and esthetics.

Fig. 4-55

References

1. McLean JW. Construction of metal ceramic bridgework. In: *Science and Art of Dental Ceramics*. Vol II. Chicago: Quintessence Publishing Company; 1980:331-354.

2. Miller LL. Framework design in ceramo-metal restorations. *Dent Clin N Amer*. 1977;21:699.

3. Sullivan D, Parel SM. *Esthetics and Osseointegration*. Chicago: OSI Publishing Company;1983:15-16.

4. Albrektsson T. Bone Tissue Response. In: Brånemark P-I, Zarb GA, Albrektsson T, eds. *Tissue Integrated Prostheses: Osseointegration in Clinical Dentistry*. Chicago: Quintessence Publishing Company; 1985:129-143.

5. Skalak R. Biomechanical considerations in osseointegrated prosthesis. *J Prosthet Dent*. 1983;49:843-848.

6. Bridger DV, Nicholls JL. Distortion of ceramo-metal fixed partial dentures during the firing cycle. *J Prosthet Dent*. 1981;45:507.

7. McLean JW. The metal ceramic veneer crown. Monograph IV *Science and Art of Dental Ceramics*. Vol 1. Chicago: Quintessence Publishing Company; 1979:273-298.

Chapter 5

A Composite of Overdenture Applications

The overdenture treatment is a good alternative to a fixed, bone-anchored prosthesis. This treatment modality offers distinct advantages to many patients who would benefit from two or three carefully placed implants. Where an unstable full denture is converted to, or replaced by, an implant-supported overdenture, function, fit and stability can be greatly improved. When two or more implants are placed, bone resorption is decreased significantly.[1]

Esthetics can be improved when soft and/or hard tissue defects exist by modifying the dimensions of the acrylic resin. Facial and lip support can be improved by these changes in the design of the prosthesis.[2,3 (pp 173-174,183-186,216-220)]

Often, economics dictate a patient's choice of treatment. Since the overdenture prosthesis requires a minimum of two implants, surgical and hardware costs are reduced.

With fewer abutments and increased access, the overdenture works well for patients with limited hygiene maintenance ability. In some cases, phonetics and speech are impaired by the space between the alveolar ridge and the fixed bone-anchored bridge. The overdenture is a good alternative when these problems are present.[4 (pp 219-225)]

In a situation where six fixtures are placed and three fail to osseointegrate, the remaining three can support an overdenture. This can work as a permanent solution or as an interim prosthesis while new implants are placed.

Hader-Retained Maxillary Overdenture Supported by Core-Vent Implants

The Core-Vent implant-supported Hader bar (APM, Stern Gold) offers many alternatives in treatment planning. It is clearly indicated where the patient does not want a fixed implant-supported bridge and feels comfortable with a clip-secured removable overdenture. The Hader system is a cost-effective treatment modality. This plan requires a minimum of two implants, in contrast to the suggested five or six implants for the traditional fixed bone-anchored bridge.

The finished Hader bar weighs approximately six to ten penny weight (Troy weight), while the traditional fixed frame is usually 20 to 30 penny weight. This system offers the option of rotation of the overdenture when the bar is fabricated straight (Figs. 5-1 and 5-2).

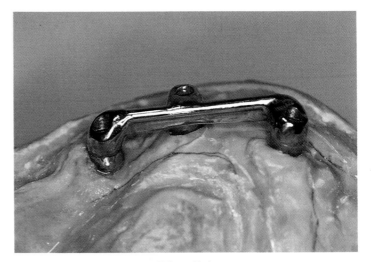

Fig. 5-1

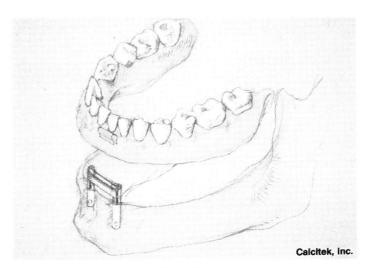

Fig. 5-2

With more than two implants and a bar that is not continuously straight, there is minimal movement, increased lateral stability and no rotation of the overdenture. The latter, however, does apply added stress to the implants and remodeling bone. The minimal vertical requirement (3.5 mm), and the fact that Core-Vent sleeves and Hader bar patterns are castable, make this combination very compatible.

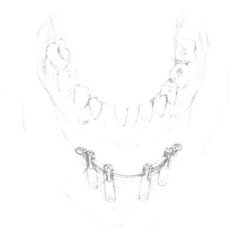

Fig. 5-3

This master cast shows three Core-Vent brass replicas in the anterior of the maxilla.

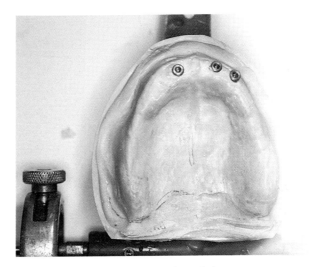

Fig. 5-4

Casts are mounted on a semi-adjustable articulator using conventional procedures.

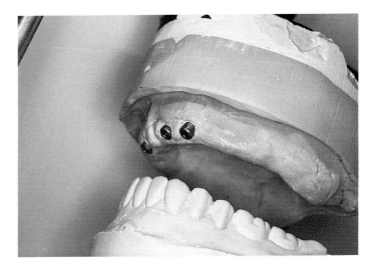

Fig. 5-5

Core-Vent components include: the brass replica (# BTF), plastic castable sleeve (# PSO), and titanium prosthetic screw (# TSF).

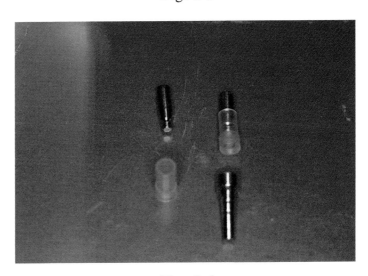

Fig. 5-6

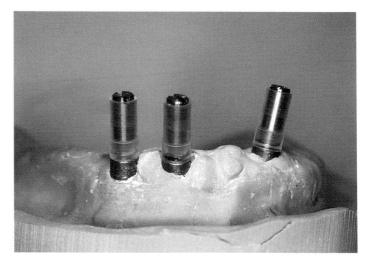

Fig. 5-7

The plastic sleeve is secured in place with titanium screw. DO NOT overtighten, as the plastic sleeves will crack.

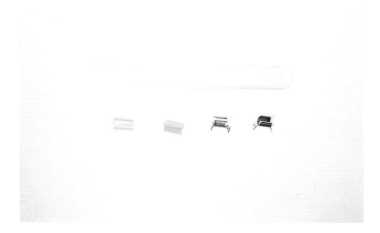

Fig. 5-8

The Hader clip bar ensemble consists of a plastic castable rider bar, plastic clips, and metal clips.

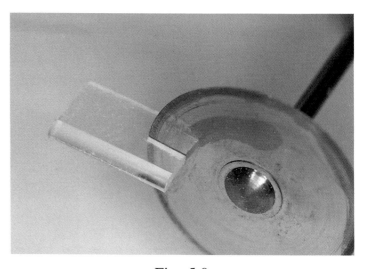

Fig. 5-9

Using the articulated counter cast as a guide, the bar is cut to the vertical height with a thin disc. The bar must not interfere with the setup or the arrangement of teeth if at all possible.

Any irregularities at the tissue level can be scalloped with a bur.

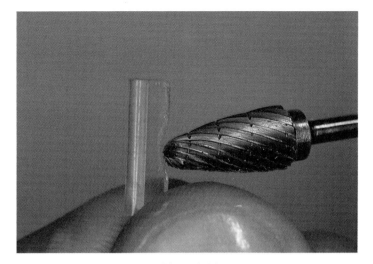

Fig. 5-10

The sized bar is placed between the plastic sleeves and held in place with utility wax. The plastic bar should be kept parallel with the ridge.

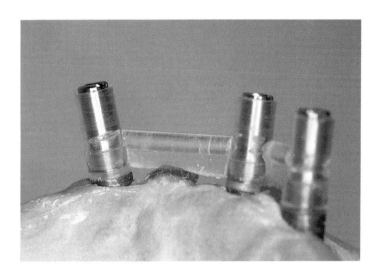

Fig. 5-11

Small increments of DuraLay are painted around the plastic sleeve incorporating the plastic bar. DO NOT allow DuraLay resin to flow beyond the margin of the plastic sleeve. After resin has polymerized, it should be smooth-finished to a thickness of 1.5 mm.

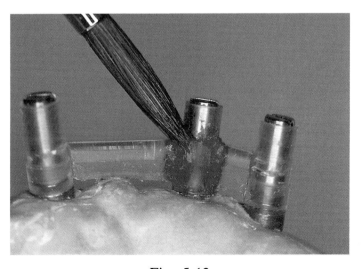

Fig. 5-12

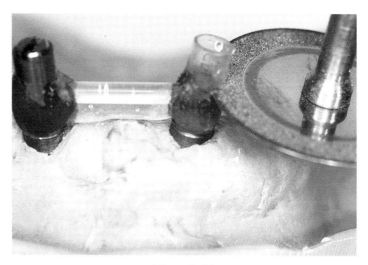

Any portion of the sleeve which now rises above the plastic Hader bar pattern should be cut level with the bar.

Fig. 5-13

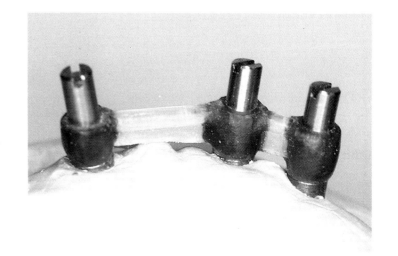

Thin areas and voids are thickened and smoothed using crown and bridge wax. When the bar-sleeve pattern is complete, it should be checked for a perfect passive fit. If each plastic sleeve does not fit with total accuracy, the offending area must be sectioned and re-attached.

Fig. 5-14

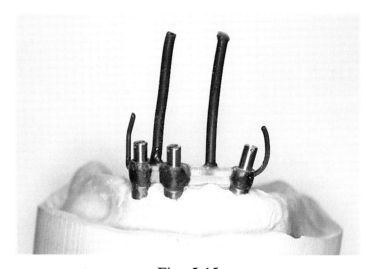

The pattern can now be sprued and readied for investing. One twelve gauge sprue between each section and an eighteen gauge closed vent sprue at each distal are adequate for successful casting. The plastic bar is now invested following recommended manufacturer's instructions for base alloy metals (Rexillium III, Jeneric Pentron).

Fig. 5-15

After casting and cooling, the bar is retrieved and sandblasted. The metal is finished and polished according to standard crown and bridge procedures.

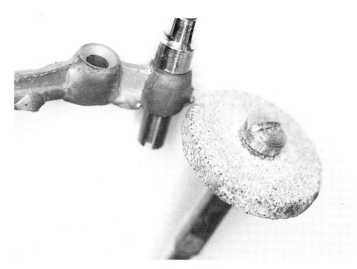

Fig. 5-16

It is recommended that brass replicas be used to protect the margins on the casting.

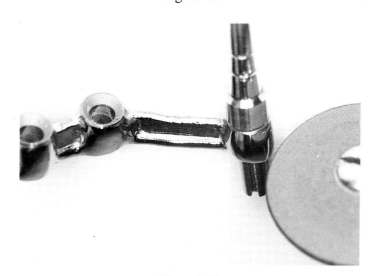

Fig. 5-17

Prosthetic screws are placed through the sleeves and secured to the cast. Using an ultra thin disc, the screws are lightly scored at the height of the sleeve. The screw is removed from the cast and cut through at this height. Since the slot for the screwdriver has been cut off, a new slot must be cut in.

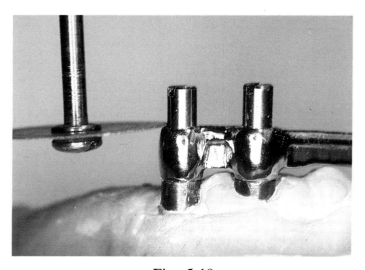

Fig. 5-18

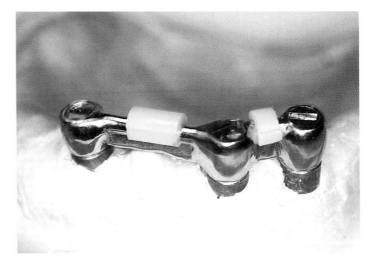

This is a view of the base alloy Core-Vent-supported Hader bar with two plastic clips.

NOTE: Sometimes the space between screws will not accommodate a full clip. The plastic clips can be cut to size.

Fig. 5-19

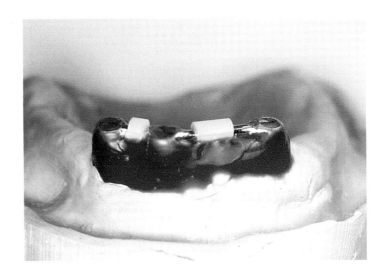

This Hader bar has plastic riders blocked out for the fabrication of a pink Triad material baseplate. The base is light cured and finished to proper peripheral borders.

Fig. 5-20

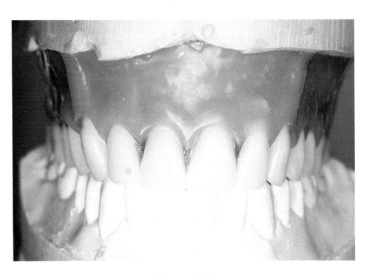

Teeth (Bioform IPN, Dentsply) are set and tried in for esthetics and occlusal harmony. The Hader bar is checked for accuracy.

Fig. 5-21

After verification of casting fit and denture setup, the restoration is flasked and boiled out in the normal manner.

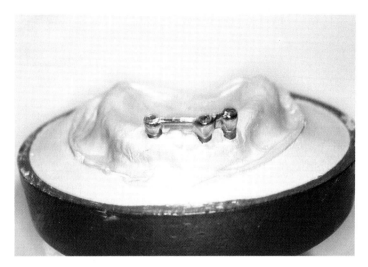

Fig. 5-22

Metal riders are chosen for the finished restoration, and two are placed in the large area of the bar. Since the metal riders cannot be shortened, no rider is placed in the smaller section.
NOTE: Plastic riders are easier to replace chairside and can be cut for smaller areas, but are not adjustable. Metal riders can be adjusted and have a longer life, but they are more difficult to replace due to their means of retention.

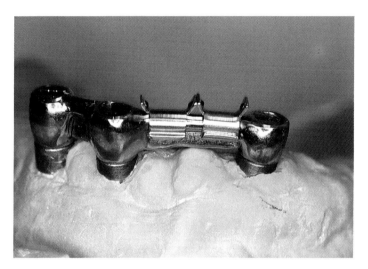

Fig. 5-23

Since the bar on the cast causes many undercuts, it is necessary to block out at this time. A mixture of one-half plaster and one-half ordinary pumice is used to facilitate an easy breakout. The plaster/pumice mix is brought at least half way up the Hader clip. This extra room will allow the clinician the needed space to adjust the clip as necessary. The cast and prepared bar are painted with a separating medium and packed in the conventional manner using Lucitone 199 and cured at 165° F for nine hours.

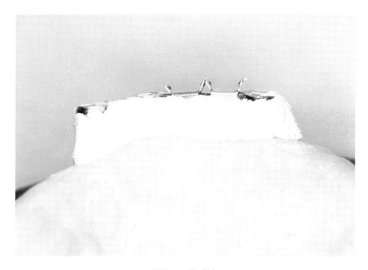

Fig. 5-24

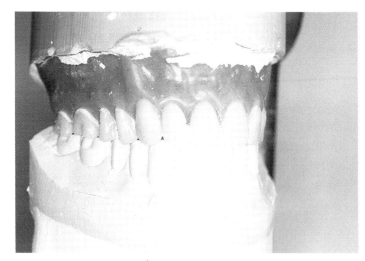

After curing, the restoration is retrieved and remounted on the articulator to refine occlusion and eliminate processing errors.

Fig. 5-25

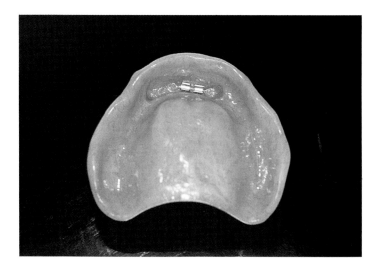

The Hader bar is carefully removed from the tissue side of the denture, and the restoration is finished and polished.

Fig. 5-26

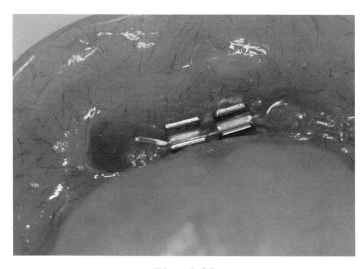

The tissue side of the denture shows two acrylic-retained metal Hader riders. Note the edge of the metal riders. The retention can be increased or reduced by adjustment with a thin instrument.

Fig. 5-27

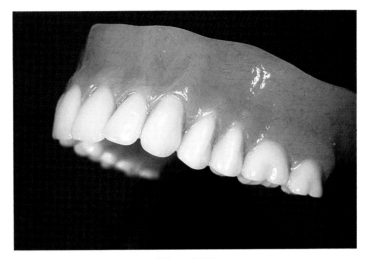

The finished Hader-retained Core-Vent implant-supported overdenture ready for delivery.

Fig. 5-28

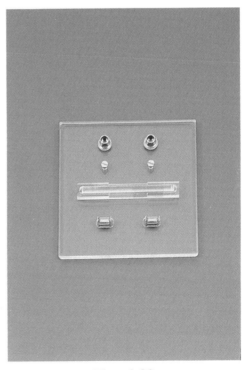

The Brånemark System Clip Bar Kit follows the same protocol as the Core-Vent System with the exception that gold cylinders are used in place of the castable sleeves and the alloy of choice must have a melting temperature below 2350° F.

Fig. 5-29

The Ball Attachment

The Nobelpharma ball attachment is for overdenture treatment on single abutments. The use of this attachment is for retention and stabilization. When used in overdentures it reduces shock, pressure and torque. It is simple to use, saves time, and is a very convenient treatment plan for the patient. The patient's existing denture can be used, or a new one fabricated. The ball attachment is screwed directly into the fixture. The attachment comes in three heights: 3 mm, 4 mm, and 5.5 mm. On top of the ball there is an internal hexagon used when installing the screw. The screw is made of pure titanium.

The diameter of the ball is 3.5 mm in this titanium ball attachment with abutment connector.

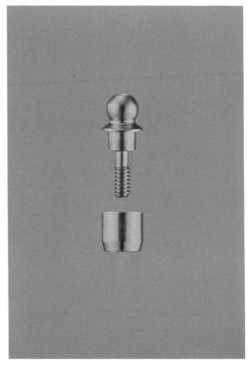

Fig. 5-30

The plastic cap has a rubber O-ring which is incorporated in the denture. O-rings have a retention capacity of 500 gms each. They can be cold cured chairside or heat cured in the laboratory.

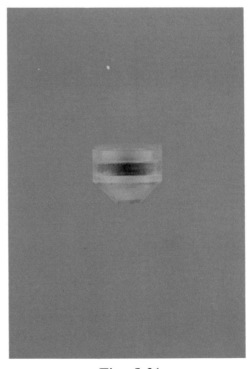

Fig. 5-31

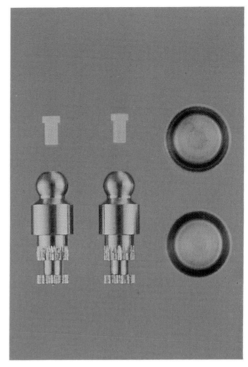

Fig. 5-32

These ball attachment brass replicas have spacers and caps with O-rings. The plastic spacer fits on top of the brass replicas during the processing procedures. The spacer is used to create the necessary room on top of the ball, permitting minor denture movement during function.

One thickness of baseplate wax is put in the area of the ball attachments in the patient's denture. The denture is seated in the patient's mouth. Using slight pressure, the positions of the ball attachments are imprinted in the wax. When the areas have been located, they are hollowed out.

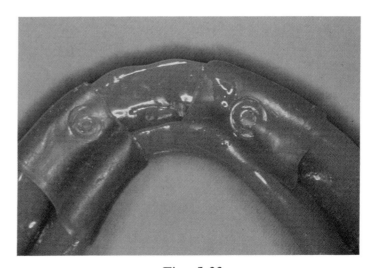

Fig. 5-33

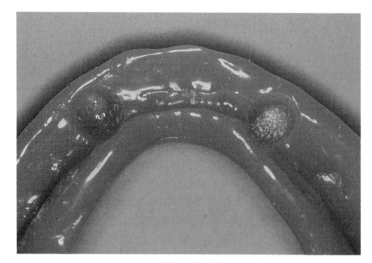

Fig. 5-34

This procedure is repeated until the denture seats to the proper position.

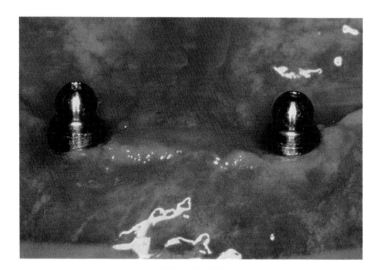

Fig. 5-35

This intraoral view shows the ball attachment.

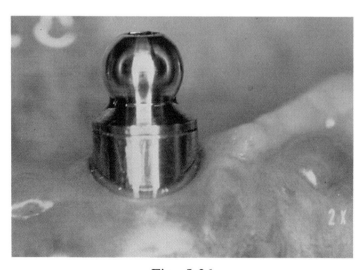

Fig. 5-36

This close-up of the ball attachment shows good tissue response and adaptation.

Acrylic is removed from the tissue side of the denture and a reline impression is taken. Brass replicas of the ball attachment are placed in the negative reproduction present in the impression. The master cast is poured and the denture and cast are mounted on a reline jig. The denture is then relined in the normal manner using Lucitone 199.

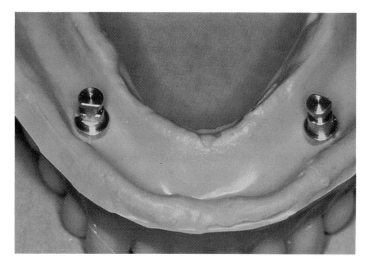

Fig. 5-37

This master cast has brass ball attachment replicas. When heat curing the female during laboratory procedures, it is necessary to block out with stone from the cast-up and around the visible part of the brass replica to the underside of the attachment. This will prevent leakage of acrylic to the inside of the plastic caps and O-ring.

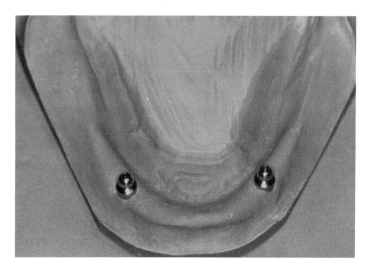

Fig. 5-38

This is a view of the tissue side of the processed denture with female O-ring attachment.

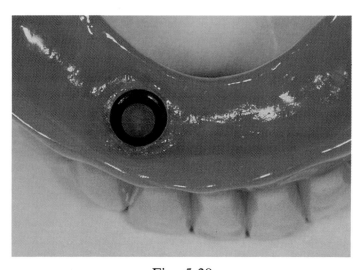

Fig. 5-39

Core-Vent Ball Attachment

Another ball-type attachment is the Core-Vent Ball Attachment. These can be screwed or cemented to the fixture. The ball attachments shown are cementable.

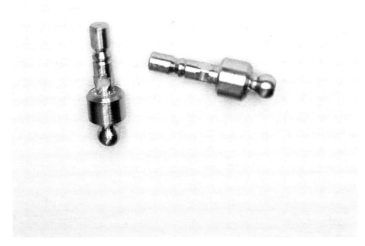

Fig. 5-40

The tissue side of the denture reveals the female housing with the O-ring. Fabricating procedures are similar to all other ball attachments.

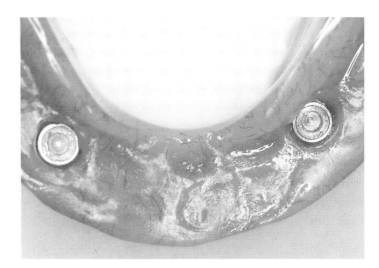

Fig. 5-41

Maxillary Overdenture with Ceka Revax Attachments Supported by Brånemark System Implants

The Ceka Revax system contains all of the components needed to produce a successful fixed/detachable overdenture. The proven record and long-term use of this attachment in the dental field makes it a familiar and viable treatment plan. The Revax system has a complete accessory armamentarium for the replacement and maintenance procedures.

The attachment from the factory has 830 grams of retentative force which can be adjusted upon patient request. This retention is well above the minimum of 400 gms per attachment advocated by Lehmann and Arnin.[5]

The overall size of the Revax (3.8 mm high and 3.4 mm wide) allows the restoration to remain within normal parameters. When the Revax is used in a substructure bar with a precision milled design, increased lateral stability is achieved.

The strength and durability of the overdenture is increased when a metal backbone or superstructure is incorporated in the prosthesis as in Figure 5-21. The Revax is available in four alloys for casting with virtually any metal.

The male attachment is preserved during processing through the use of duplicate processing pieces. After processing, finishing, and polishing, Ceka-Bond cement should be applied to the male threads before they are screwed into the female. This prevents the male spring pin from unthreading during function. However, the male spring pin may still be removed at any time using the special tool.

This maxillary bite rim has incorporated Brånemark System impression copings. The design is both implant and tissue borne.

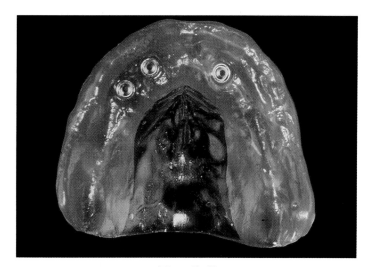

Fig. 5-42

Side view of mounted casts illustrates the amount of labial ridge and tooth contour that must be restored to produce a true skeletal Class I occlusal scheme.

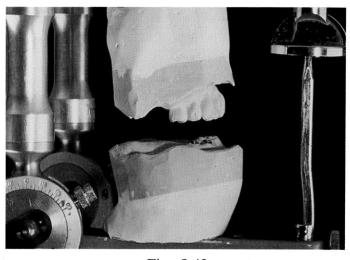

Fig. 5-43

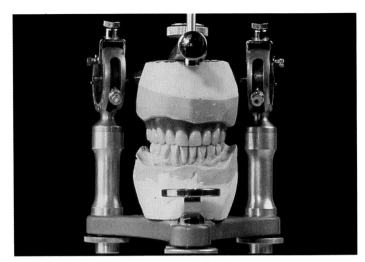

Teeth are selected (Vita Lumin Acryl) and set up in Class I position for a diagnostic evaluation.

Fig. 5-44

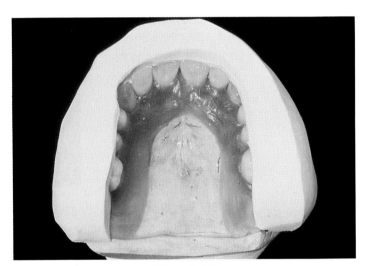

The master cast is indexed, lubricated, and a silicone matrix (Nobelpharma) applied.

Fig. 5-45

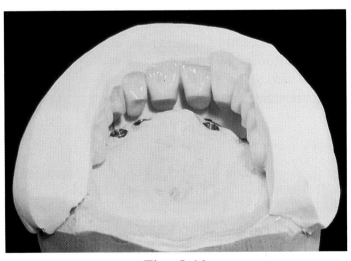

All pink wax is steam cleaned away. The master cast supports matrix with teeth held in setup position.

Fig. 5-46

This diagram shows the implants and the proposed design of the substructure bar with Revax-retained overdenture.

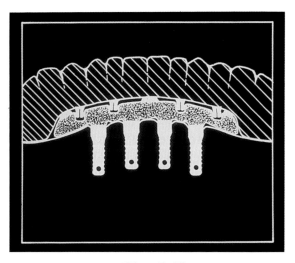

Fig. 5-47

The arrows pointing at the bar indicate raised milled platforms. This design allows room for attachment function and supports vertical forces with the tripod effect. The four recessed slots on the top of the bar represent the Revax finale patterns.

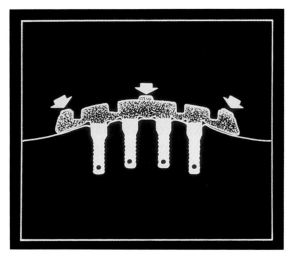

Fig. 5-48

The entire bar pattern must combine all attachments, raised platforms and exterior surfaces into a precision milled path of insertion.

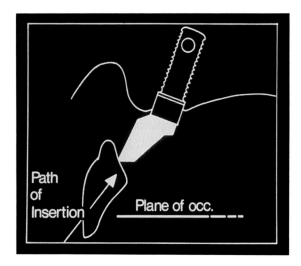

Fig. 5-49

The matrix is checked on the master cast. Teeth are ground out to make room for the bar attachment.

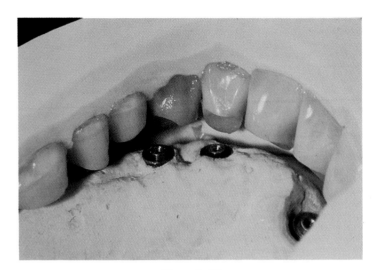

Fig. 5-50

A bar is fabricated using castable plastic cylinders and self-cure resin. The Revax females are positioned with a paralleling mandril in arrangement with the path of insertion and secured with resin.

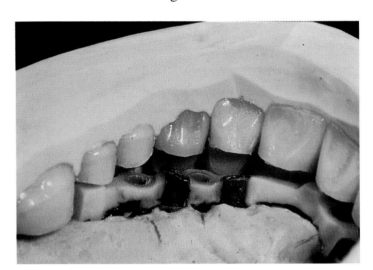

Fig. 5-51

In this occlusal view of the completed substructure bar pattern, the spruing, investing and casting techniques all follow the protocol in Chapter 3.

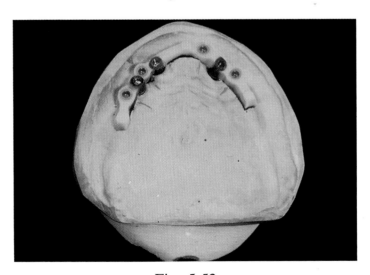

Fig. 5-52

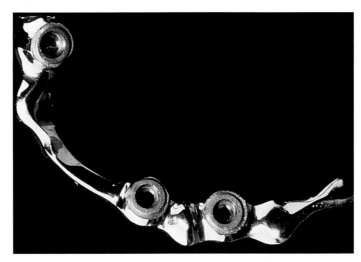

Cast cylinders are protected during all finishing and polishing procedures with metal protective caps.

Fig. 5-53

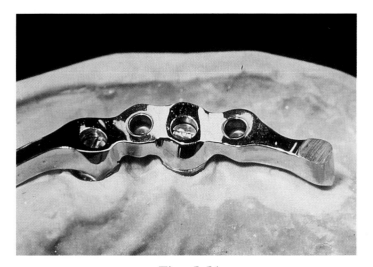

The finished and polished bar is secured to the master cast with gold screws. Note the Revax females, distal platform, and parallel lingual wall.

Fig. 5-54

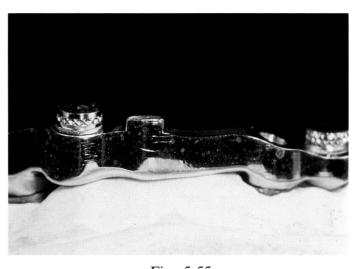

A labial view of the gold bar with Revax males in place.

Fig. 5-55

An intraoral view of the substructure bar try-in.

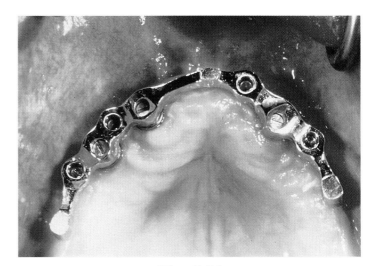

Fig. 5-56

The lubricated bar is shown with processing pieces in place over a silicone blockout. The red outline on the cast indicates the proposed border of the blockout material.

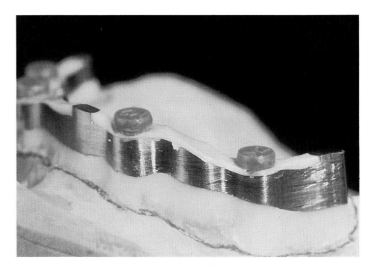

Fig. 5-57

An impression is taken of the entire cast with bar. A refractory model is then poured.

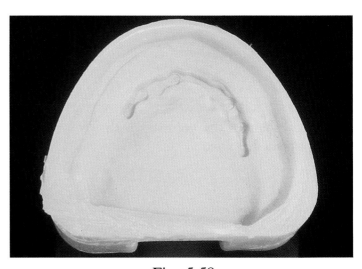

Fig. 5-58

The superstructure pattern is created on the refractory cast. Care is taken to keep the pattern thin in areas contacting the teeth in the matrix. The cast with completed pattern is sprued, invested, burned out, and cast in a type IV gold alloy.

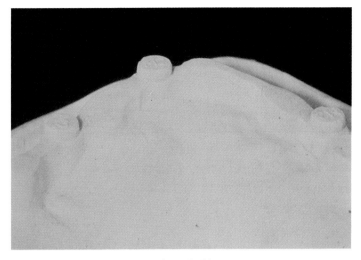

Fig. 5-59

The casting is devested, cleaned, and finished. All areas that have tissue contact are highly polished.

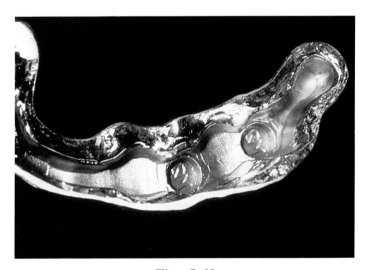

Fig. 5-60

The overcasting is fitted to the bar on the master cast and checked with the tooth matrix. All final adjustments in the metal frame and acrylic teeth are made at this time.

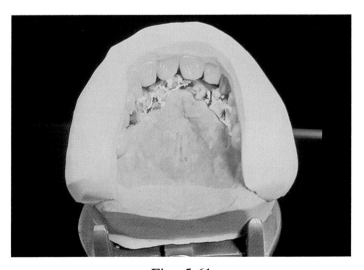

Fig. 5-61

Using the matrix, denture teeth are luted to the overcasting and master cast. Peripheral borders are finished in wax, with the lingual aspect in a horseshoe design. Investing, processing and finishing techniques are completed as per Chapter 3. With care, the master cast can be preserved.

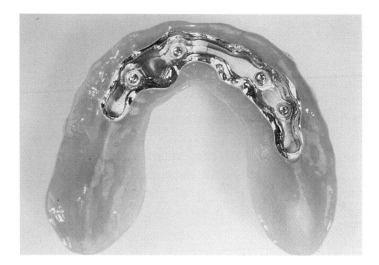

Fig. 5-62

The occlusal view shows the finished prosthesis with polished rugae adding to the correct anatomical features.

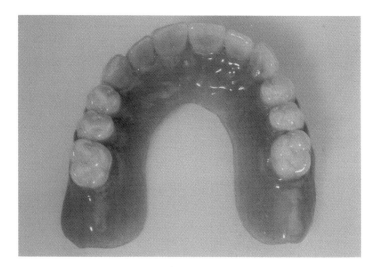

Fig. 5-63

The final delivery of bar and overdenture. Meticulous laboratory fabrication should make this a relatively uncomplicated procedure.

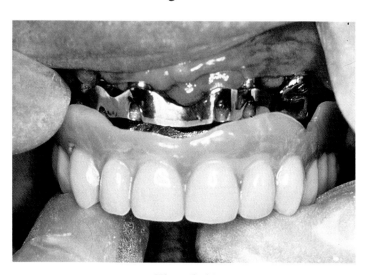

Fig. 5-64

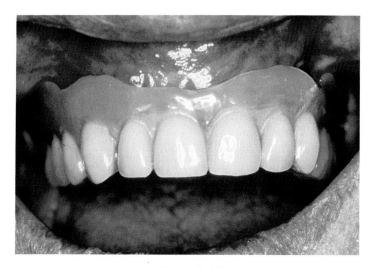

The labial flange effectively masks the metal bar. Correct selection and placement of teeth combine to make this a very esthetic restoration.

Fig. 5-65

Mandibular Overdenture Retained by Shiner Magnets

The components to augment the Shiner magnets are listed from left: keeper replica for mast cast; processing piece; impression piece; and metal o-ring spacer.

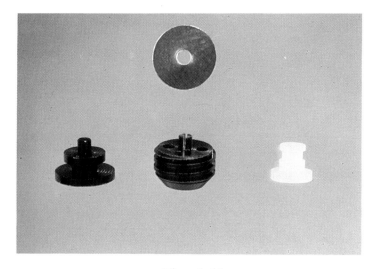

Fig. 5-66

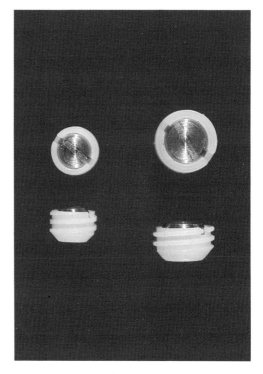

Fig. 5-67

The Shiner mini magnets are on the left and the regular size are on the right. The mini size measures 2.4 mm vertically and 3.9 mm in diameter. The regular size is 3.4 mm in height and 5.5 mm in diameter.

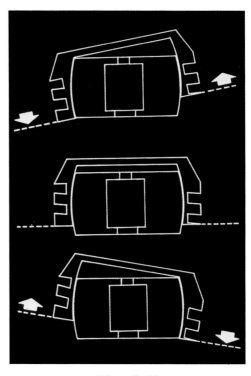

Fig. 5-68

The action between the actual magnet and the housing allows slight movement of the prosthesis. The magnet remains connected to the keeper, which eliminates air gaps and the "snap back" effect.

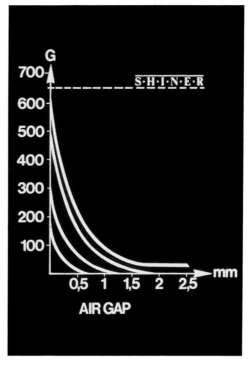

This graph illustrates how the loss of intimate contact between magnet and keeper diminishes available retention.

Fig. 5-69

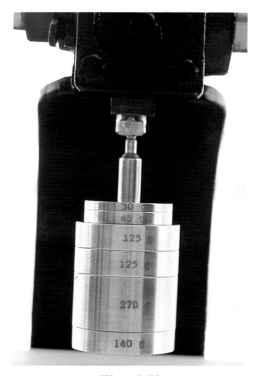

This test instrument indicates that the Shiner regular magnet can hold 1.5 lbs of weight bars. The mini size has approximately 30% less retention.

Fig. 5-70

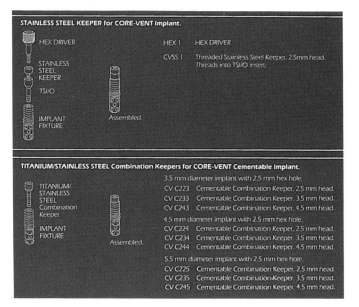

The top portion of the diagram illustrates the complete armamentarium for the Core-Vent threaded stainless steel keeper system. The bottom half shows titanium stainless steel keepers for the Core-Vent cementable system.

Fig. 5-71

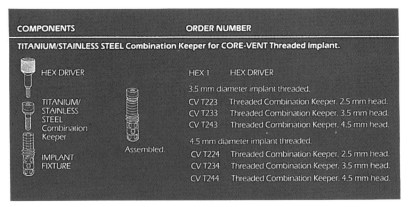

Fig. 5-72

Components and part numbers are shown for the titanium stainless steel keepers in the Core-Vent threaded system.

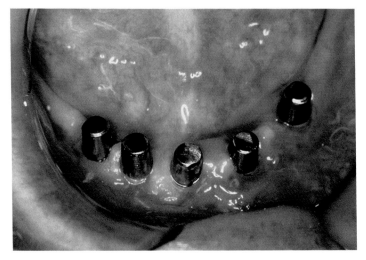

Healing abutments are secured to osseointegrated fixtures during the interim period.

Fig. 5-73

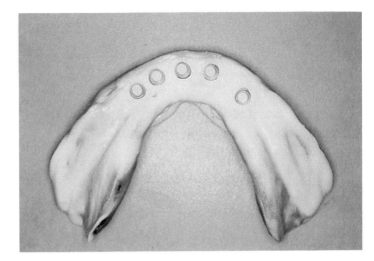

Fig. 5-74

The patient's existing denture is modified by removing acrylic from the tissue side to accept the five healing abutments. A soft liner material (Coe Super Soft, Coe Inc.) is used to refit the denture to the abutments.

A hex driver is secured to the titanium stainless steel combination keeper.

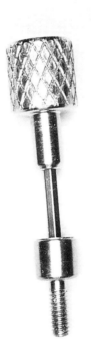

Fig. 5-75

Keepers are screwed into fixtures with perio-pack around the perimeter to aid in tissue healing.

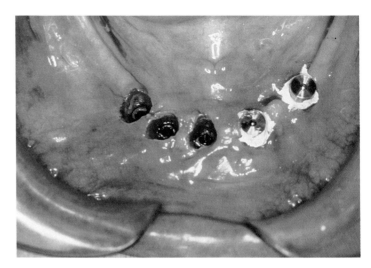

Fig. 5-76

All keepers are secured to implant fixtures with the hex driver and checked clinically and radiographically for fit.

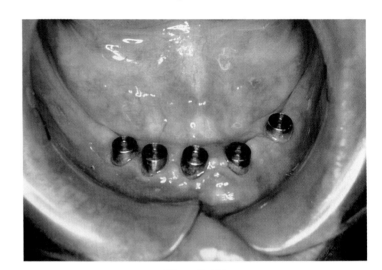

Fig. 5-77

Impression pieces are secured to keepers using the center hole plug.

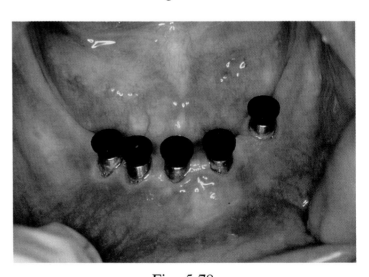

Fig. 5-78

The outer rim of the keeper matches perfectly with the impression coping. The two components are held together with a pressure fit. The intimate fit between these two components is a check point for total accuracy.

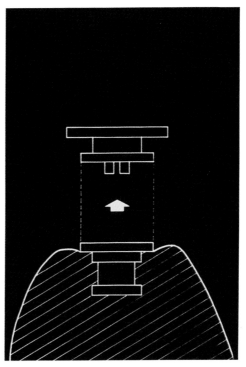

Fig. 5-79

This master cast has the keeper replicas intact. All replicas must be cleaned and air dried for maximum retention of black processing males.

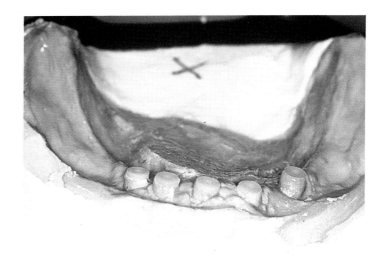

Fig. 5-80

Black processing males are placed; teeth are selected (Bioform IPN, Dentsply Int.); and a full wax setup is completed. Usually the teeth in the areas of the magnets must be hollow ground.

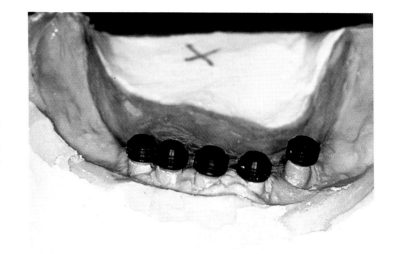

Fig. 5-81

After the wax try-in has been verified, it is then flasked and boiled out in the usual manner.

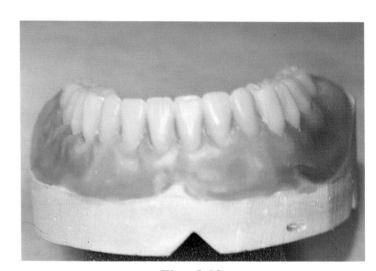

Fig. 5-82

After boil-out, the processing male at the top is seated down over the o-ring spacer to the keeper replica in the master cast. This metal spacer provides room for the clinician to adjust the position of the magnet as needed. The restoration is now packed with Lucitone 199.

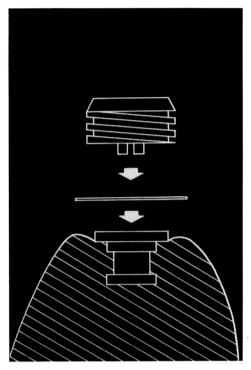

Fig. 5-83

This is a view of the finished and polished overdenture with the processing males intact. Note the appearance of the acrylic at the junction of the attachment.

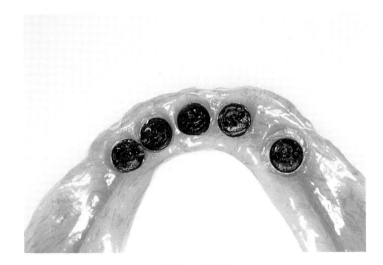

Fig. 5-84

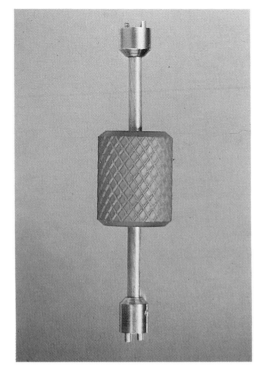

Fig. 5-85

This metal tool has a magnet hole configuration at one end and processing piece prongs at the other.

Only after the prosthesis is completely polished should the males be carefully backed out with the metal tool.

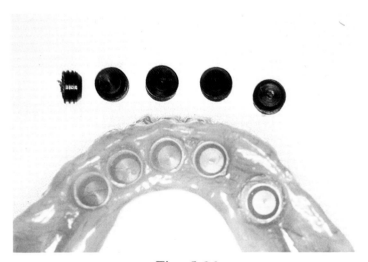

Fig. 5-86

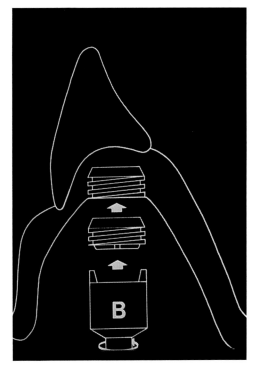

This schematic diagram shows the magnet driver, magnet, and matching void created by the processing piece.

Fig. 5-87

Magnets are carefully screwed into threaded sites. Do not force the magnet into the socket. If it does not screw in easily, it must be backed out and started again.

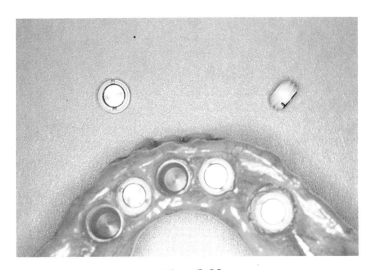

Fig. 5-88

The finished magnet-retained overdenture with all components in place.

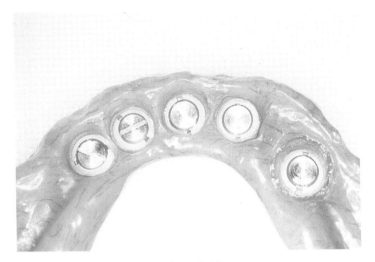

Fig. 5-89

The intimate fit of the magnets to the keepers is imperative. Pressure indicator paste (Mizzy Inc.) is applied to the magnets and checked intraorally. Magnets can be adjusted to attain perfect magnet-to-keeper fit.

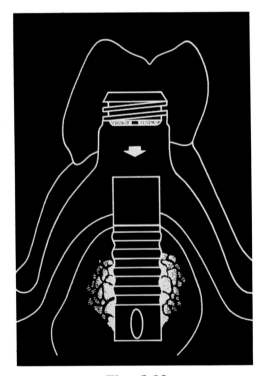

Fig. 5-90

The finished and polished magnet-retained overdenture.

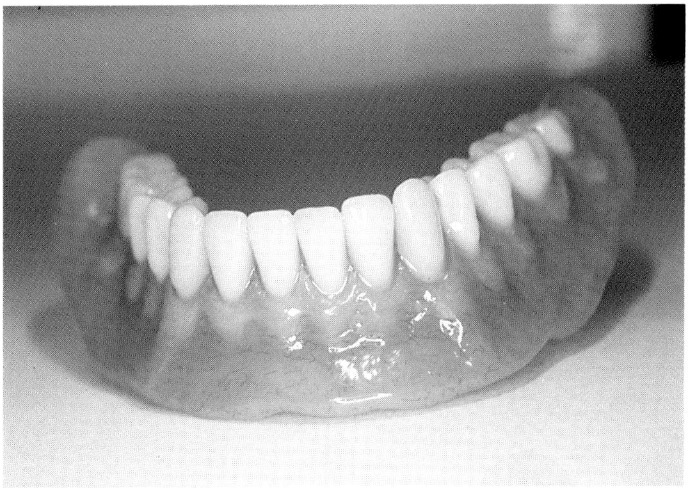

Fig. 5-91

References

1. Zarb GA, Jansson T, Jempt T. Other prosthodontic applications. In: Brånemark P-I, Zarb GA, Albrektsson T, eds. *Tissue Integrated Prostheses: Osseointegration in Clinical Dentistry*. Chicago: Quintessence Publishing Company; 1985:283-287.

2. Parel SM. Implants and overdentures: the osseointegrated approach with conventional and compromised applications. *Int J Oral Maxillofac Imp*. 1986;1:93-99.

3. Albrektsson T, Zarb GA. *The Brånemark Osseointegrated Implant*. Chicago: Quintessence Publishing Company; 1981.

4. Lehmann KM, Arnim FV. Studies on the retention forces of snap-on attachments. *Quint Dent Tech*. 1978;7:45-48.

Chapter 6

Single Tooth Abutment

The single tooth abutment is based upon a non-rotational component which fits directly to the hexagonal head of an osseointegrated implant fixture.[1] This component eliminates the trans-epithelial connector, while using the abutment screw for final fixation. The component is augmented with impression copings that fit the hex of the implant and fixture replicas with the hex portion that is reproduced to maintain the spacial relationships of the components during fabrication.

Inter-occlusal space often plays a major part in the selection of abutments. The most adaptable and versatile abutment for very restricted working areas is the castable plastic UCLA abutment made by 3-I Company. Using this component, the technician can create many important changes in design which overcome difficult challenges in esthetics. The correct casting procedures and metal finishing techniques are critical factors in the success of this restoration (Figures 6-4,5,6). The integrity of the internal hex lock portion of this casting must be perfectly maintained. The Brånemark System single tooth abutment is a non-rotational titanium component that precisely engages the titanium osseointegrated implant fixture. This maintains the ideal harmony of a titanium interface.[2] This abutment is available in five different tissue depths (Figure 6-15) and offers the option of a cementable sleeve or a direct cast restoration.

Gold alloy single tooth cylinders from the 3-I Company (Figure 6-3) have a machined hex lock that exhibits an excellent predictable fit to the hexagonal fixture. Two abutment screws are included with the cylinder: the actual fixation screw; and a long laboratory screw that is useful in forming the substructure pattern as well as the access hole. Careful investing and casting procedures do not adversely affect the fit of this component.

Brånemark System hex lock gold cylinders are supported by a special hexagonal titanium abutment and abutment screw. This cylinder is secured by a small gold screw, thus preserving the original design feature of the weak link being the prosthetic gold screw. A regular laboratory guide pin is used for fabrication techniques (Figures 6-54 and 6-55).

Another type of single tooth abutment from Core-Vent features a titanium cementable post or a plastic castable post pattern. Working from a master cast containing a fixture replica, the post pattern is seated firmly in place. Either post can be modified to create the unique dimensions required for each different application. For complete adaptability, the castable post is more versatile. The finished implant-supported post abutment is then cemented and an impression taken. The new master cast is very similar to a Pindex crown and bridge format. The single tooth restoration is fabricated using the pattern material, metal alloy, and veneer material of choice. The completed crown is now cemented to the implant post abutment.

The Brånemark System angulated abutment gold cylinder can also be used in special single tooth situations. The screw-retained cylinder is altered (Figures 6-38 and 6-39). to create a fixed screw post design. The definitive crown is then built on traditional crown and bridge principles and cemented over the fixed screw post abutment.

The UCLA Abutment

A master cast with fixture replica (3-I Co., #ILA20) in place. Soft material (Coltene G-mask, Coltene, Inc.) is applied to the area surrounding the implant to simulate the soft tissue response.

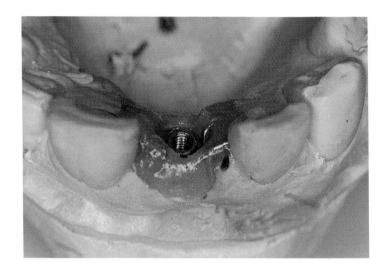

Fig. 6-1

A lingual view shows the height of the tissue labial to the fixture replica. To duplicate the correct sagittal profile of the tooth, this area must be treated with great care in both metal design and ceramic crown contour.

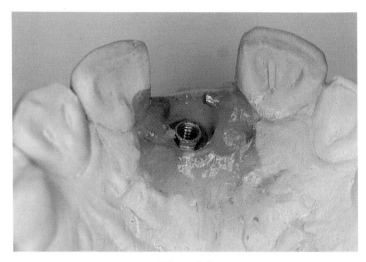

Fig. 6-2

Components include at top: abutment screw with gold UCLA hex lock abutment (3-I Co.,   GUCA 1), abutment screw and castable hex lock UCLA abutment (3-I Co., UCLA B1) and Brånemark System fixture.

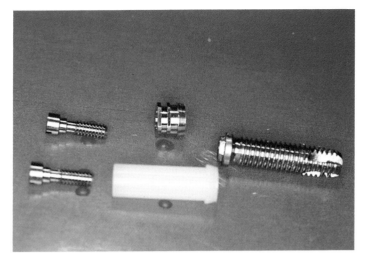

Fig. 6-3

Crown and bridge wax is added to the adjusted UCLA pattern to form the desired substructure contours. The pattern is sprued and invested in a high heat phosphorous investment (Ceramigold II, Whip Mix Corp). The ring is burned out and cast in a high noble ceramic alloy (Eclipse, J. M. Ney Co.).

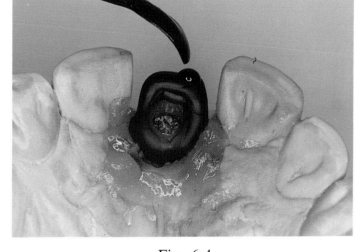

Fig. 6-4

The lapping mandril, diamond paste, and the centering sleeve are shown here. The cast abutment pattern must be finished prior to veneer application with this system. The mandril is placed in an ordinary handpiece, with the casting being held to the smaller end with the centering sleeve. The paste is applied to the flat surface of the mandril and ground against the margin of the casting. This creates a milled interface surface which contacts the implant with greater accuracy.

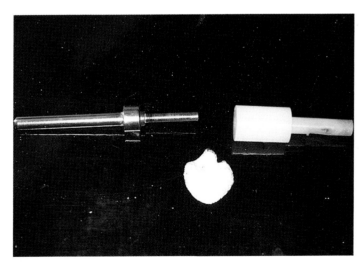

Fig. 6-5

The metal substructure is shown fastened to the titanium implant fixture. This technique enables the technician to verify the marginal fit of the casting.

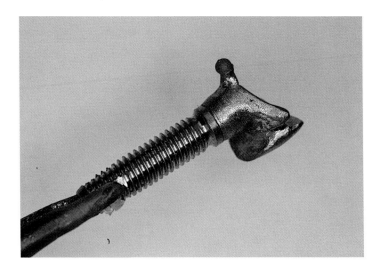

Fig. 6-6

This lingual view shows the casting when seated on the fixture replica. Note the good cervical contour and sufficient incisal support.

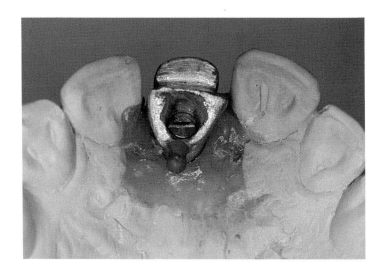

Fig. 6-7

The metal pattern after degassing and opaque application. The internal portion of the abutment must be cleaned of all porcelain particles before firing.

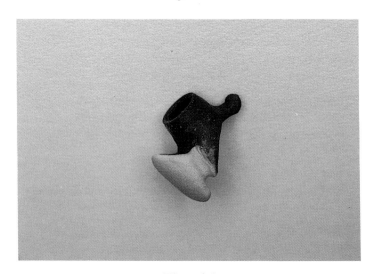

Fig. 6-8

The body and incisal porcelain powders are built up on the model. Labial and incisal length contours are over-built to allow for condensing and shrinkage (Figures 6-9 and 6-10).

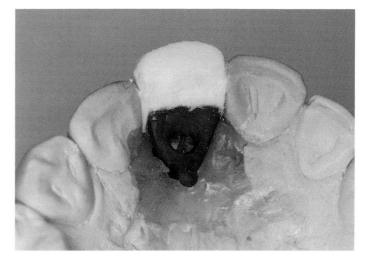

Fig. 6-9

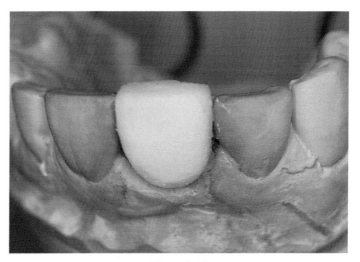

Fig. 6-10

The abutment crown is removed and final porcelain additions are completed.

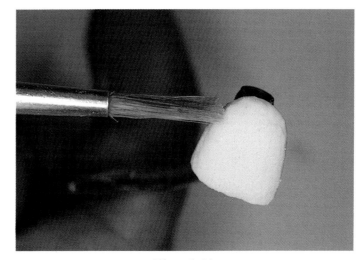

Fig. 6-11

The porcelain as it appears after the first bake.

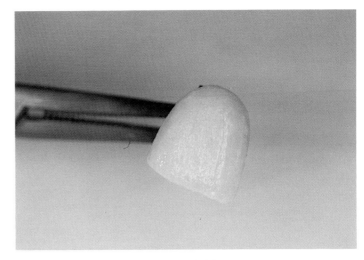

Fig. 6-12

Final glazing and polishing are complete. The restoration allows for natural tooth characteristics without compromising the desired esthetics.

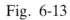

Fig. 6-13

The Brånemark System Titanium Single Tooth Abutment

The single tooth abutment developed by Nobelpharma Inc. has six components. In the column at right the fixation screw at the top (DCA #090) secures the abutment in the center (DCA #088) to the implant. In the left hand column a laboratory guide pin at top attaches the impression coping (DCA 099) in the center to a fixture replica (DCA 084).

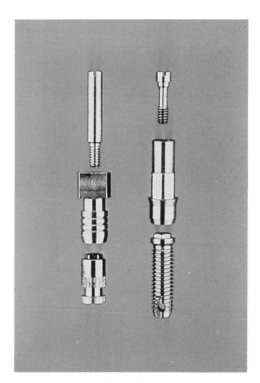

Fig. 6-14

The abutment comes in five lengths for different tissue depths (1 mm-DCA 085; 2 mm-DCA 086; 3 mm-DCA 087; 4 mm-DCA 088; and 5 mm-DCA 089). The abutment has a maximum diameter of 5 mm at the margin of the shelf. The crown is built up above this margin.

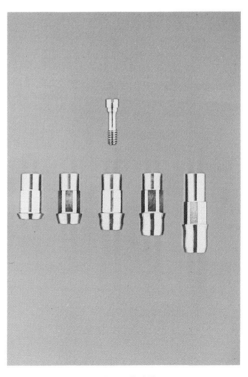

Fig. 6-15

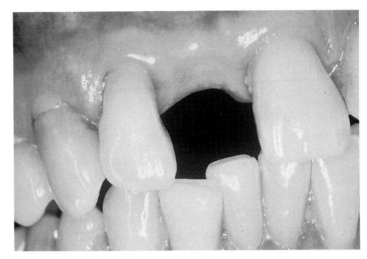

Fig. 6-16

This patient shows attractive healthy dentition demanding a very esthetic restoration.

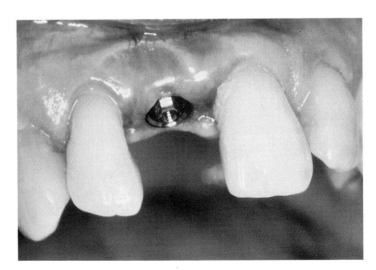

Fig. 6-17

The fixture placement and angulation are excellent.

The diagram shows the impression coping with the guide pin. Sometimes it is necessary to reduce the width of the impression coping to fit a small inter-tooth space.

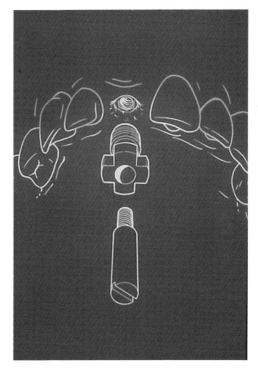

Fig. 6-18

The interface between implant and impression coping must be clean and tight to insure accurate pickup.

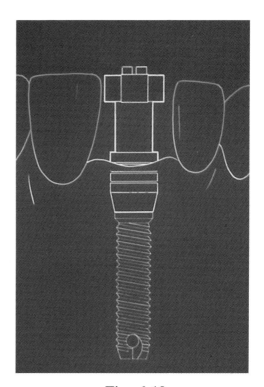

Fig. 6-19

After impression material has set, self-cure resin is added to the impression tray and connected to the impression coping. This is done to stabilize the coping within the impression. Care is taken not to cover the screw slot with the resin.

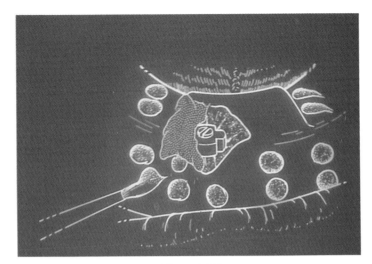

Fig. 6-20

The completed impression.

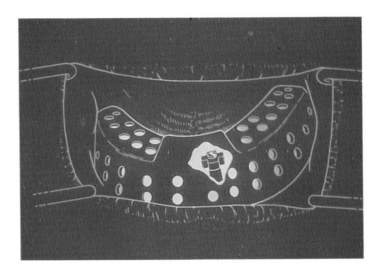

Fig. 6-21

Close inspection of the impression reveals the good detail of the soft tissue and the clean coping surface. A wax block-out is used on the exposed metal neck of the impression coping to facilitate easy separation from the master cast.

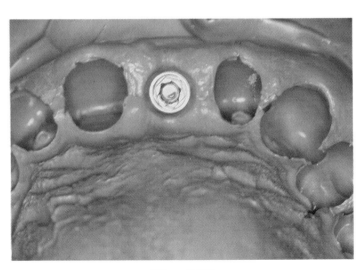

Fig. 6-22

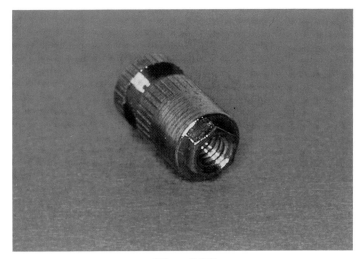

Fig. 6-23

This close-up shows how the fixture replica duplicates the hexagonal head and internal screw threads of the implant.

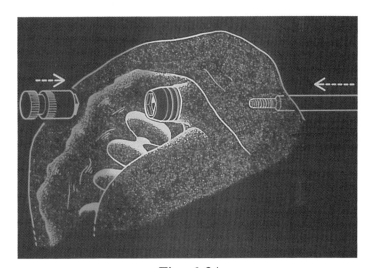

Fig. 6-24

The laboratory guide pin attaches the fixture replica to the impression coping. The master cast can now be poured.

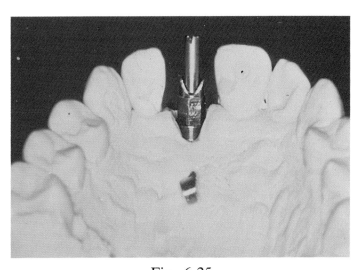

Fig. 6-25

Metal is reduced from the single tooth abutment to allow room for occlusal clearance.

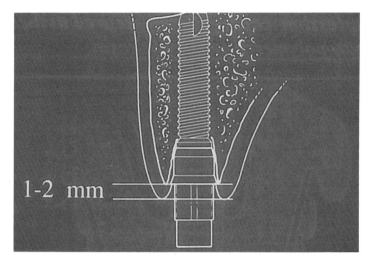

Fig. 6-26

When selecting the single tooth abutment, it is important that the crown margin extend 2 mm below the gingiva.

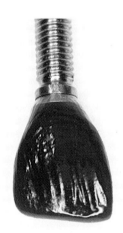

The pattern is waxed to full contour and cut back.

Fig. 6-27

This cross section illustrates the optimum relationship of contour and fit.

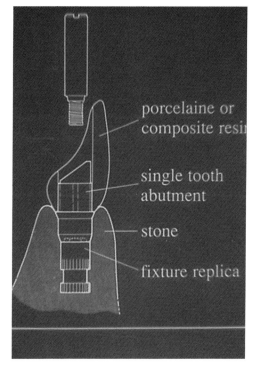

Fig. 6-28

The metal pattern finished to the titanium abutment shows excellent marginal fit.

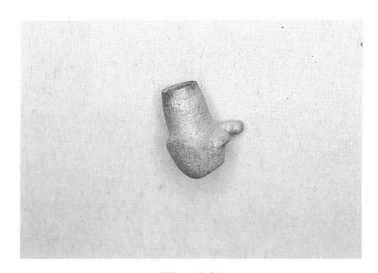

Fig. 6-29

The ceramo-metal sleeve is degassed, opaqued, and readied for porcelain application.

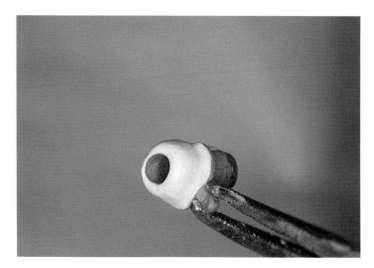

Fig. 6-30

The porcelain is built up in the normal manner.

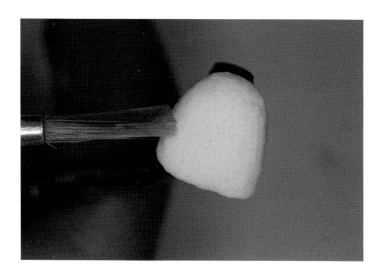

Fig. 6-31

The porcelain is carefully finished and glazed. The ceramic crown can now be cemented to the single tooth abutment.

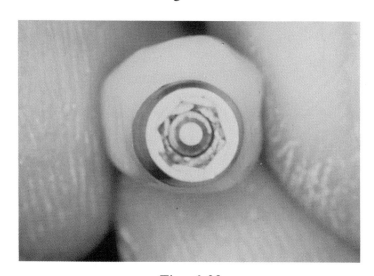

Fig. 6-32

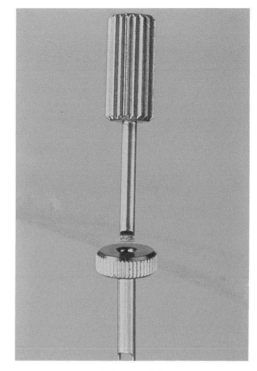

The screwdriver (DIA 253) has an anti-rotational mechanism (DIA 252) which allows the slot head to tighten the screws while the implant is stabilized.

Fig. 6-33

The single tooth abutment is seated for try-in.

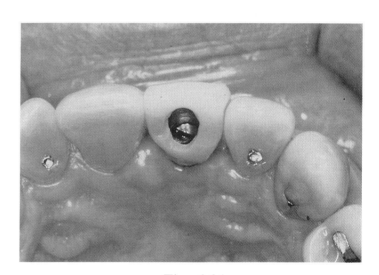

Fig. 6-34

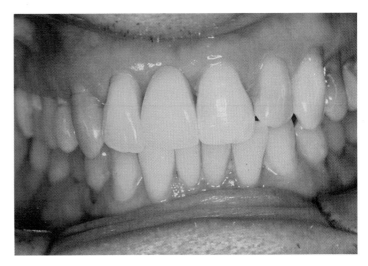

Lip retractors reveal good soft tissue adaptation and shade match.

Fig. 6-35

Correct anatomy creates a harmonious relationship between the single tooth replacement and the natural teeth, forming a normal smile line.

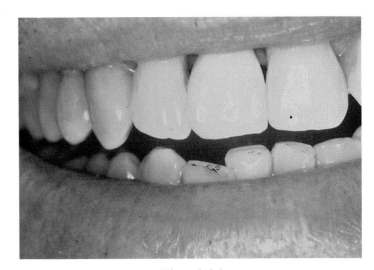

Fig. 6-36

BRÅNEMARK SYSTEM MODIFICATION

Angulated abutment for single tooth application

A master cast with a Brånemark System angulated abutment in the area of the maxillary right canine. After articulation, it was evident that the fixture placement and angulation would prevent standard procedures from achieving an acceptable esthetic result.

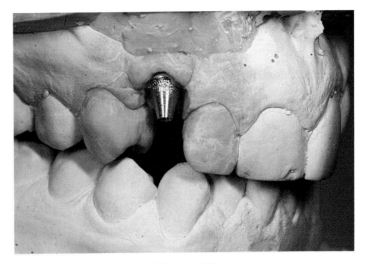

Fig. 6-37

An angulated gold cylinder is used to accept gold solder, creating a screw-fastened post and core.

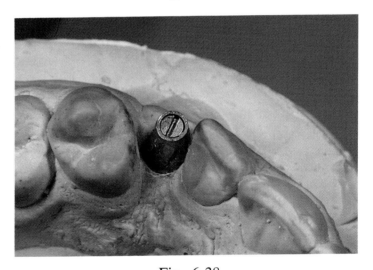

Fig. 6-38

A cylinder post with overcasting. Note the retention grooves cut into the axial walls of the post and the lingual holding button on the overcasting.

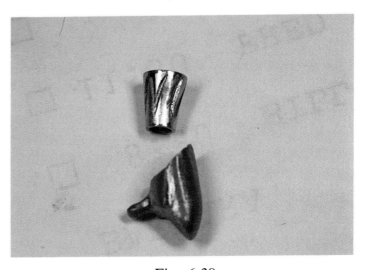

Fig. 6-39

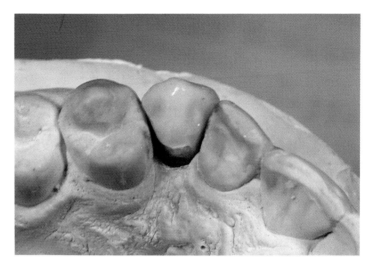

An occlusal-lingual view of the finished crown shows good mesial and
distal contact, along with developed
lingual anatomy.

Fig. 6-40

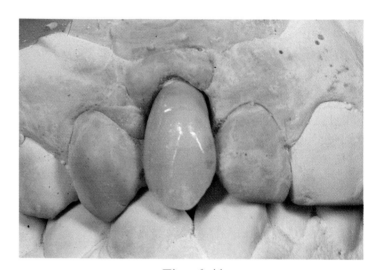

This labial view illustrates shade-
modified ceramics on the cervical
areas and the restored normal buccal
contour.

Fig. 6-41

The Brånemark System CeraOne Abutment

The CeraOne Abutment and gold abutment screw is designed to accept a cementable
ceramic core restoration. The ceramic cap is made from densely sintered aluminum oxide
(99.7% Al2 O3). With no metal core, the esthetic capabilities are increased. The short
cap measures 5.8 mm in height with a .7 mm thickness. The tapered long ceramic cap
is useful in anterior applications.

The components and hardware for this system include from left and top to bottom: impression coping, abutment replica and healing cap, gold abutment screw, abutment, titanium fixture, cut down coping, aluminum oxide ceramic core, aluminum oxide ceramic core for anterior.

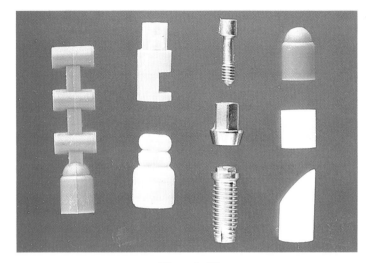

Fig. 6-42

The abutments come in five heights: 1 mm; 2 mm; 3 mm; 4 mm; 5 mm. The Nobelpharma Torque Controller,™ shown previously in Figure 6-53, has a setting to screw the gold abutment screw with a force of 32 N cm.

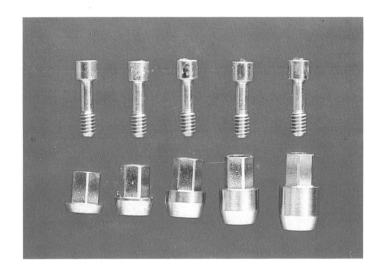

Fig. 6-43

The abutment and gold screw are placed intraorally.

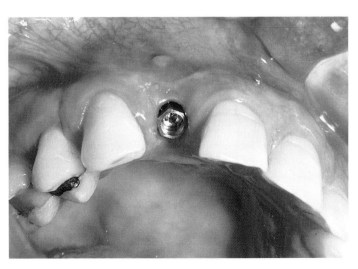

Fig. 6-44

A radiograph verifies the accurate placement of the abutment.

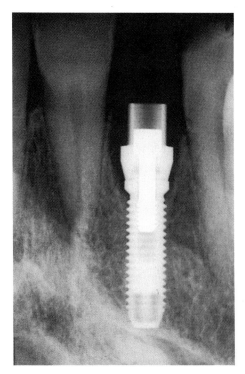

Fig. 6-45

The plastic impression coping is placed intraorally with a friction fit.

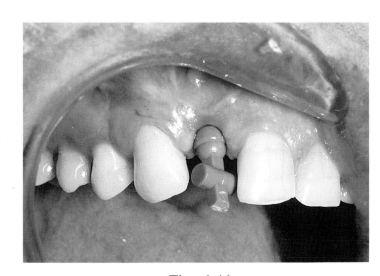

Fig. 6-46

A conventional impression is taken and the impression coping is incorporated. It is recommended that a heavy-bodied impression material be used.

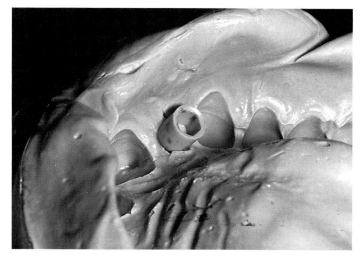

Fig. 6-47

The plastic yellow abutment replica is carefully placed into the female portion of the impression coping.

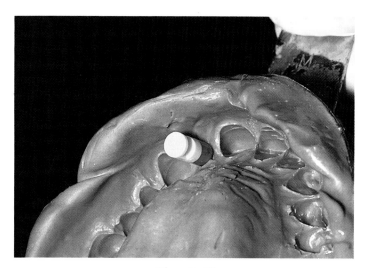

Fig. 6-48

Soft tissue material is placed around the gingival area of the crown prototype. The model is then poured in improved die stone. A ceramic cap is placed onto the abutment replica, and the restoration is now ready for buildup.

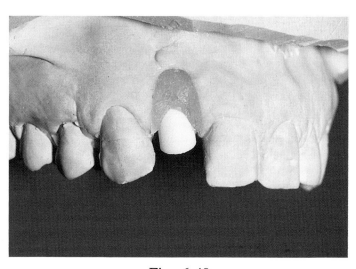

Fig. 6-49

Porcelain is applied according to the special instructions, removed from the master cast, and final contours added as needed. The porcelain must be of a type intended for all-porcelain crowns.

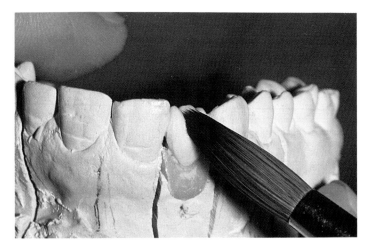

Fig. 6-50

The porcelain should be worked on wet and never allowed to dry out, to avoid porosity. A relatively slow firing cycle should be used. Prolonged firing under vacuum should be avoided.

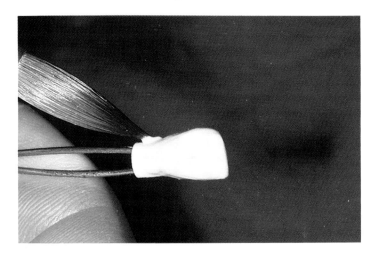

Fig. 6-51

The vacuum must be broken when the aluminum oxide-reinforced porcelain reaches the recommended firing temperature. After this has been achieved, the aluminum oxide crown can be fired at atmospheric pressure.

1. **Firing scheme for the core material**

   Starting temperature of the oven: 600° C.

   Preheating time: more than 4 min.

   Temperature rise: 55° C/min, 600-1070° C under vacuum; 55° C/min, 1070-1110° C under atmospheric pressure.

   Firing: 2 min at 1110° C under atmospheric pressure.

2. **Firing scheme for dentin material**

   Starting temperature of the oven: 600° C.

   Preheating time: more than 4 min.

   Temperature rise: 55° C/min, 600-960° C under vacuum.

   Firing: under atmospheric pressure 1 min at 960° C.

3. **Glazing**

Starting temperature of the oven: 600° C.

Preheating time: 4 min.

Temperature rise: 80° C/min, 600-920° C.

Firing: 1 min.

Use a diamond tool if it is necessary to grind the porcelain caps. The caps should be washed in a solution of diluted hydrofloric acid for five minutes, then steam cleaned or cleansed in an ultrasonic bath. The porcelain caps should be dried in air before firing.

The finished crown on abutment replicas.

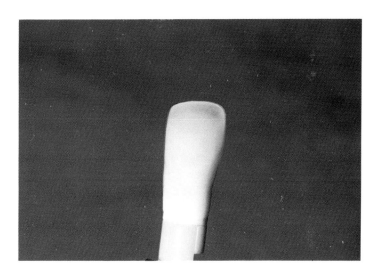

Fig. 6-52

The finished crown cemented to place. Note the superior vitality and translucency that can be attained when the metal core is eliminated.

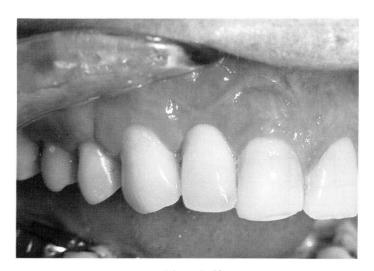

Fig. 6-53

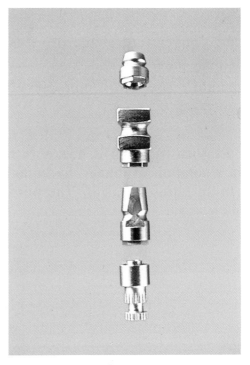

Components for the Brånemark System hex lock gold cylinder are as follows from the top: gold cylinder, square impression coping, tapered impression coping and brass replica.

Fig. 6-54

Brånemark System hex lock gold cylinders are supported by a special hexagonal titanium abutment and abutment screw. This cylinder is secured by a small gold screw, thus preserving the original design feature of the weak link being the prosthetic gold screw. A regular laboratory guide pin is used for fabrication techniques.

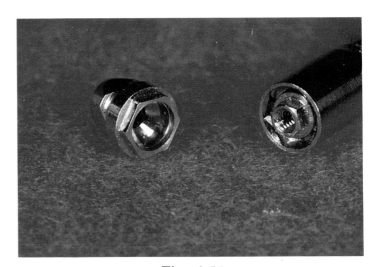

Fig. 6-55

References

1. Jempt T. Modified single and short-spanned restorations supported by osseointegrated fixtures in the partially edentulous jaw. *J Pros Dent.* 1986;2:243-248.
2. Brånemark PI, et al. Osseointegrated titanium implants in the rehabilitation of the edentulous patient. *Adv Bio Mader.* 1982;4:133-141.

Chapter 7

The Slant-Lock Retention System

The Slant-Lock System is marketed as the first system which gives the stability of a screw-retained fixed bridge and the benefits of a removable prosthesis. Since the overdenture is removable by the patient, the substructure bar and cylinders, as well as the surrounding tissue area, are easily accessible for hygiene maintenance. This is a good treatment plan for patients with limited manual dexterity. As in other overdenture applications, the fully extended denture base can replace lost bone and tissue. An important consideration is the vertical dimension. The latch and housing must be placed below the cervical of the prosthetic teeth to achieve the proper esthetic results. Space requirements can be determined after the initial wax setup and fabrication of the matrix are complete.

In a maxillary restoration, the Slant-Lock gives the esthetics of a denture flange and the support of a full natural lip contour. This system solves the phonetic problem of air passage or hissing that is sometimes present with the fixed denture bridge format.

The wax setup must be anatomically correct. Any deviation in thickness or contour of the base will put the latch in an incorrect or possibly undesirable position.

This mandibular master cast has five Brånemark fixture replicas.

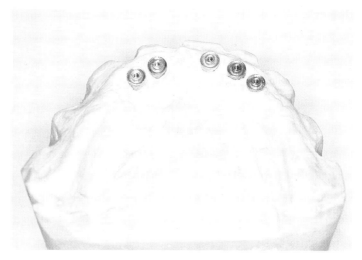

Fig. 7-1

Denture teeth are selected (Bio-blend IPN, Dentsply) and a wax set-up is completed. The master cast is keyed and lubricated in preparation for a matrix.

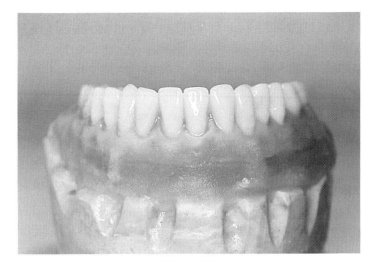

Fig. 7-2

Ramitek material is mixed and the matrix is formed.

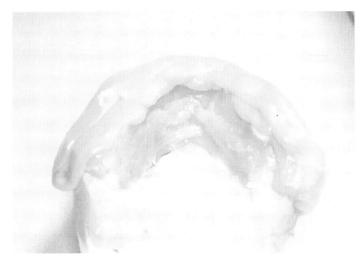

Fig. 7-3

The wax setup is removed from the cast and the general area of the latch is determined and marked. The implant spacing is a general indicator of where to place the latch. The optimal placement of the latch is in the anterior region. The prosthetic teeth must be above the position of the latch.

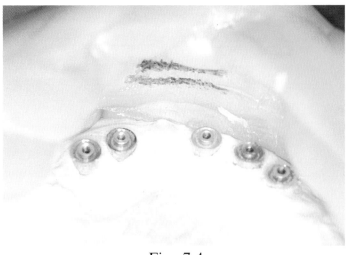

Fig. 7-4

The castable components include from the top: cylinder with adjustable runner bar, female attachment, male attachment; occlusal view of the same attachments: latch bar, regular cylinder with bar.

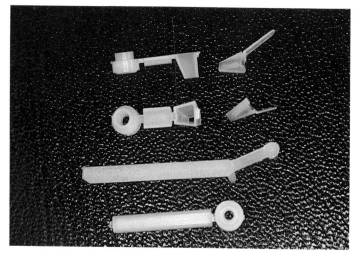

Fig. 7-5

The metal components from the top: latch housing, latch, paralleling mandril.

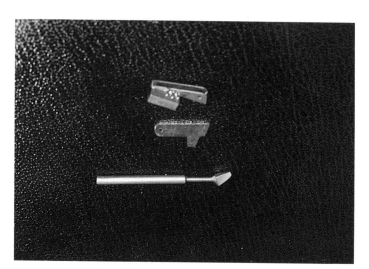

Fig. 7-6

The cast is mounted on a surveying table with fixture replicas horizontally level and as vertically parallel as possible. Lightly screw the female attachment cylinder into place, leaving room for adjustment. Place the female runner bar attachment on the ridge. The paralleling mandril is placed in the surveying arm (J. M. Ney Co.) and then in the attachment. Plastic gates can be bent to adjust the angle of the pattern to the cast. Tighten the guide pin to secure the loose plastic cylinder, and recheck the mandril.
NOTE: Do not overtighten guide pins.

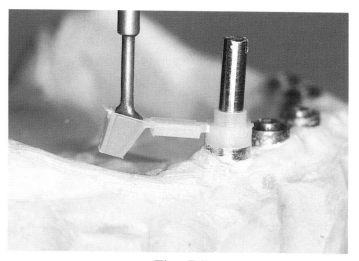

Fig. 7-7

After the position is satisfied, Zapit is used to secure all bendable parts of this runner bar. Do not allow Zapit to enter the female portion of this attachment.

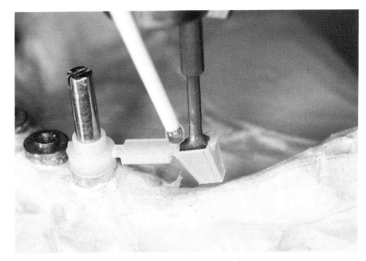

Fig. 7-8

The remaining cylinders with bars are loosely secured with guide pins. The predetermined area for the latch bar is kept open.

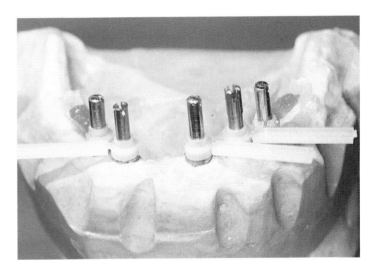

Fig. 7-9

Using a heated razor knife, the bars are cut to fit between each cylinder.

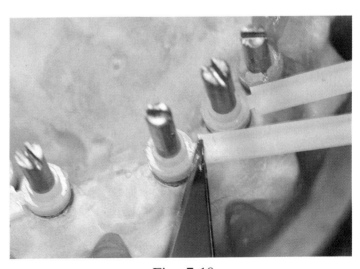

Fig. 7-10

Guide pins are tightened on each cylinder and luted together with Zapit.

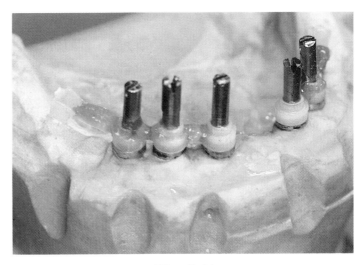

Fig. 7-11

The latch bar is designed to be square except for a 15° slant on the lingual aspect. The 15° side is marked, since after the holding tab is cut off, it is difficult to determine the difference between the labial and lingual.

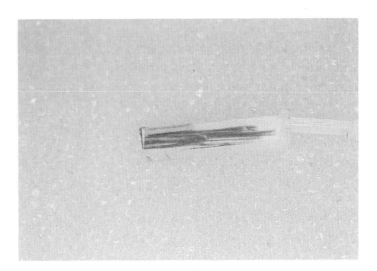

Fig. 7-12

The latch bar is placed and measured to size. The bar should extend the entire width of the cylinders in the labial position.

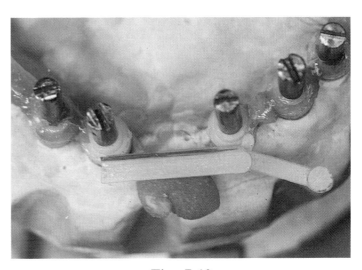

Fig. 7-13

The bar is cut to correct size.

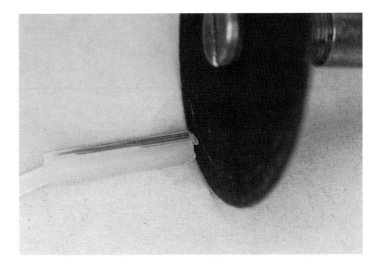

Fig. 7-14

The latch bar with metal housing and latch is held in place with utility wax. The bar must be kept in a level position. The matrix is placed on the master cast and the position of the latch bar and housing is checked for accuracy. The latch must touch the labial portion of the matrix and in the area of the mark. When the position is correct, the bar is secured with Zapit.

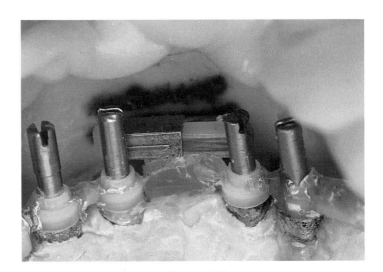

Fig. 7-15

The utility wax and latch housing are removed. The bar is waxed to final contour with a slight occlusal taper to accept the overcasting.

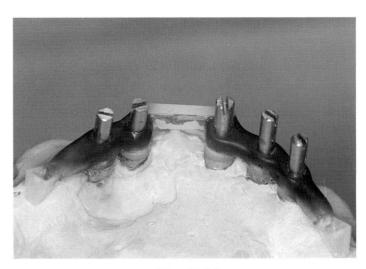

Fig. 7-16

A labial view of the completed bar. Spruing, investing and casting procedures are carried out. A base metal alloy (Rex III, Jeneric-Pentron) is used.

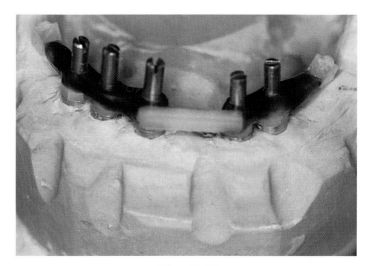

Fig. 7-17

The casting is then devested and cleaned following the protocol described in Chapter 3.

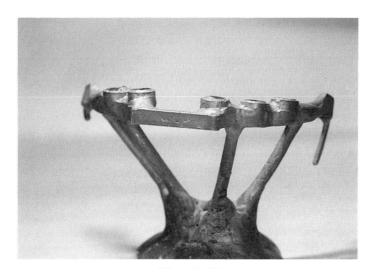

Fig. 7-18

The undercasting is finished and polished. Minimal polishing should be done in the area of the latch bar, as this is geared to fit the housing for the locking latch.

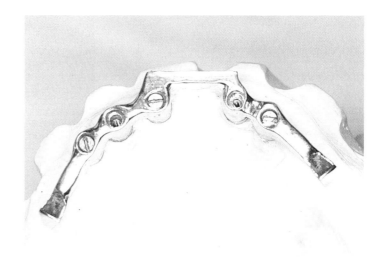

Fig. 7-19

The distal male attachments should now be fitted to their female counterpart. Any descrepancies should be relieved until the males seat securely. The overcasting is ready to be fabricated. The screw access holes are filled in level with utility wax. The distal male attachments are placed, and the Slant-Lock housing is put into the proper position.

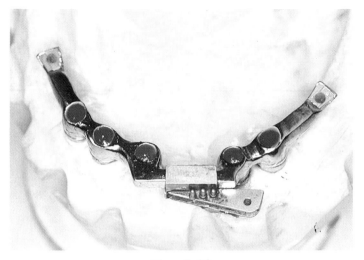

Fig. 7-20

Soft DuraLay is used to incorporate the distal male attachments and the Slant-Lock housing. When the mix of DuraLay can be hand manipulated, it is molded over and around the remaining parts of the bar. Care should be taken not to engage the undercuts of the primary bar. Soft excess DuraLay can be trimmed with a sharp scalpel-type knife. After the DuraLay has set, the overcasting must be carefully removed from the substructure. Any irregularity that prevents the frame from seating or releasing from the primary bar must now be eliminated.

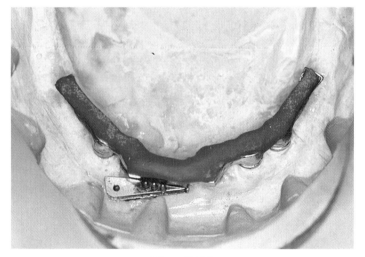

Fig. 7-21

The overcasting is sprued, invested and cast in the same alloy as the substructure bar. The temporary retention wings are waxed in for framework stabilization during investing and packing procedures.

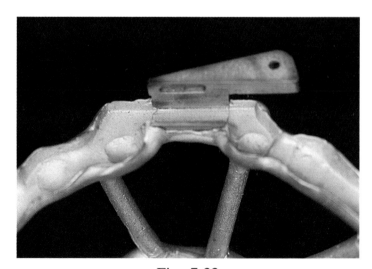

Fig. 7-22

The overcasting is diamond finished after the fit to the substructure bar has been satisfied.

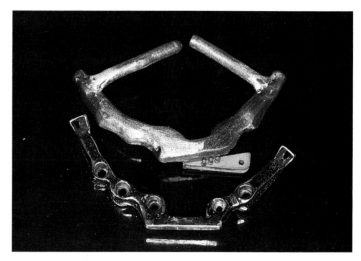

Fig. 7-23

Using the matrix, the denture teeth are set into the model with the substructure bar and overcasting in place. If possible, another try-in to verify esthetics and occlusion should be performed at this time.

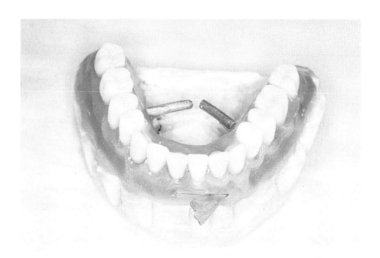

Fig. 7-24

A close-up view of the latch in the anterior section of the wax-up. If it is necessary for esthetics, the latch can be silicoated and opaqued to match the pink acrylic.

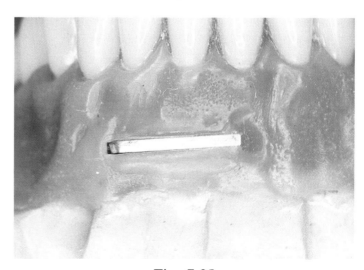

Fig. 7-25

The denture is flasked in the conventional manner and boiled out. Any undercuts in or around the substructure bar and overcasting should be blocked out at this time.

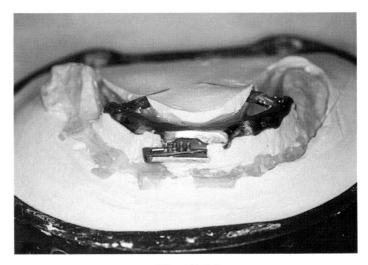

Fig. 7-26

This lingual view illustrates the temporary retention wings embedded in stone, securing the overcasting to the substructure bar during the packing procedure. The restoration is now packed in the normal manner.

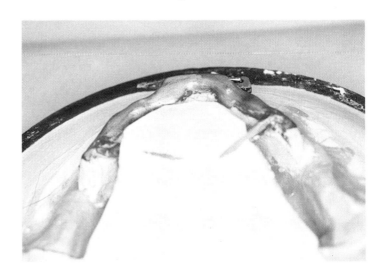

Fig. 7-27

The processed denture is carefully devested and removed from the master cast. It is then finished and polished. A facial view of the restoration with the substructure bar is shown.

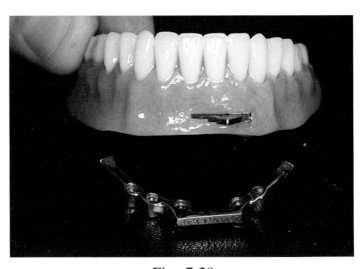

Fig. 7-28

An internal view shows the metal overstructure incorporated in the processed acrylic.

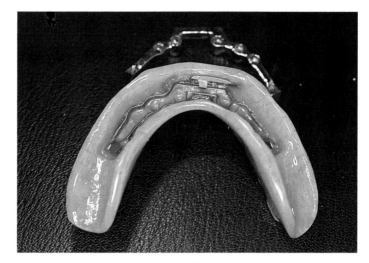

Fig. 7-29

A lingual view with the retention wings cut and polished.

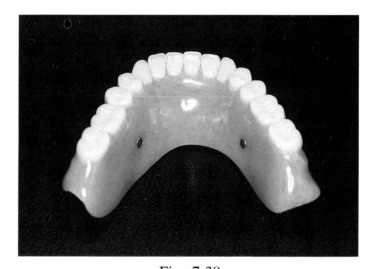

Fig. 7-30

The prosthesis is illustrated with the Slant-Lock in open position ready for insertion.

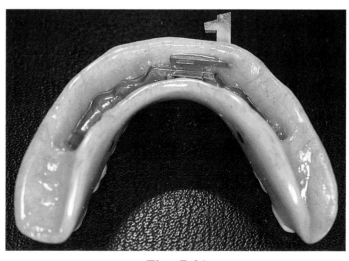

Fig. 7-31

Chapter 8

The Carbon Fiber-Reinforced Acrylic Bridge

A carbon fiber frame (currently in development by Nobelpharma AB), may offer the patient a new concept in osseointegrated restorations. This new material is designed to substitute for the metal portion of the implant-supported substructure. The metal casting is eliminated, in addition to all metal finishing and polishing procedures. This material is much lighter than metal and is very easy to work with, especially after it is cured. The carbon fiber frame might be a good alternative where allergic reactions are a concern. It should be noted that this technique is still experimental and testing is in progress. Long-term clinical results are as yet unproven.

The clinical steps when installing a carbon fiber-reinforced acrylic bridge are the same as those used for tissue-integrated bridges with metal frameworks:

1. A working model is produced using a suitable impression.
2. A bite template is produced according to specifications.
3. The clinician checks connections and performs jaw registration.
4. An acrylic (Kerr Fastcure, Romulus MI) pattern is manufactured and the teeth are set up in wax for a try-in.
5. After the try-in is tested and accepted by the clinician and the patient, the carbon fiber frame is ready to be fabricated.

   NOTE: Hand creams containing silicone grease must not be used while working with the type of heat-polymerized acrylic which is used in the bridge framework.

Carbon Fiber-Reinforced Bridge

A working model is poured using a suitable impression. An acrylic pattern is fabricated for the setting of teeth.

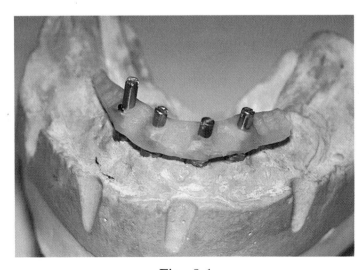

Fig. 8-1

At right: brass replica, titanium cylinder and laboratory guide pin. Components assembled at left.

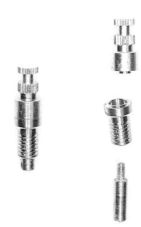

Fig. 8-2

Myerson (Myerson, Nobelpharma Inc.) teeth are set in Class I occlusion. The master cast is deemed accurate and the patient has accepted the esthetics.

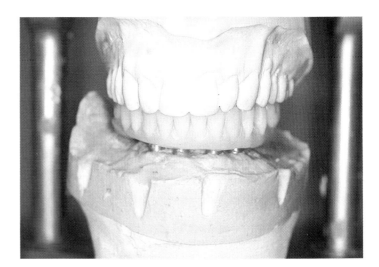

Fig. 8-3

Master cast with trial setup in indexed and lubricated to receive a silicone matrix.

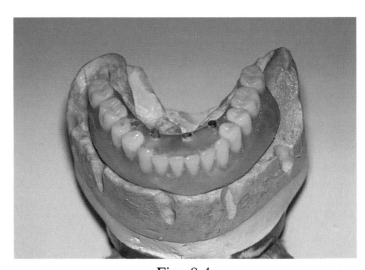

Fig. 8-4

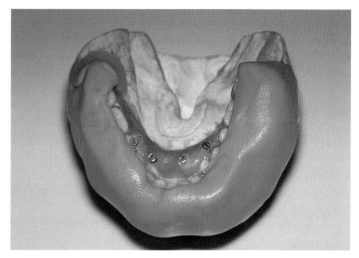

Fig. 8-5

A silicone matrix is made of the trial setup (Polysil Putty, Accurate Set Inc.).

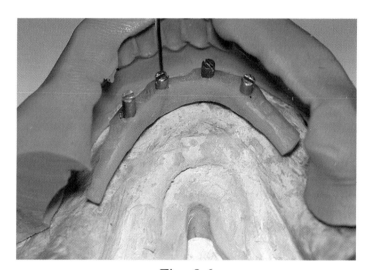

Fig. 8-6

The teeth are removed and the matrix is placed back on the cast. The acrylic frame is checked for dimensional accuracy. A 3.5 mm to 4.0 mm width and 6.0 mm height is recommended, along with a 13.0 mm distal cantilever. The actual height is 4.0 mm at the final frame finish.

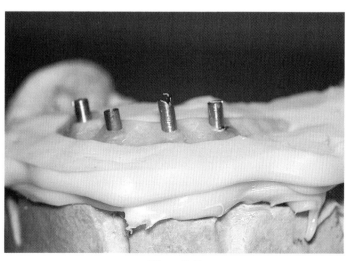

Fig. 8-7

With the frame dimensions verified, a new matrix is fabricated with Ramitek (Ramitek, ESPE Inc.). The acrylic frame is surrounded lingually and buccally, pressing the material beneath the frame and around the abutment replicas. The top is left uncovered. When the matrix has set, a razor knife is used to cut the Ramitek flush with the top of the acrylic frame. The master cast is now separated from the articular mounting disk.

Half of a denture flask is filled with plaster, and the master cast with acrylic frame is embedded, bringing the plaster to the top of the Ramitek matrix.

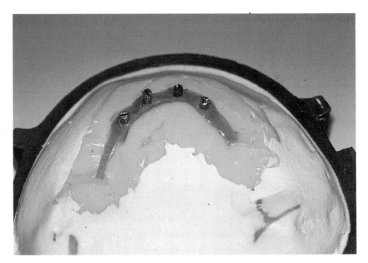

Fig. 8-8

When the plaster has set, a new 4.0 mm to 5.0 mm cap of Ramitek is placed on top of the acrylic frame to obtain a lid. The lid is pressed down onto the frame so that the guide pins leave visible impressions without penetrating the Ramitek.

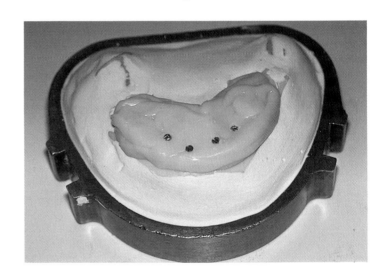

Fig. 8-9

The second half of the flask is prepared in the usual manner, assembled, filled with plaster, and closed.

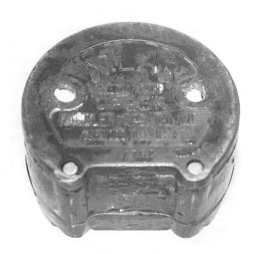

Fig. 8-10

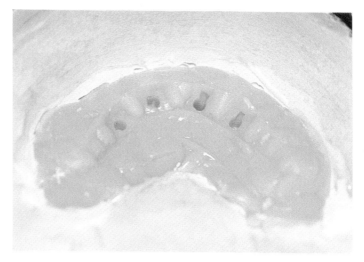

When the plaster has set, the flask is split. It is normally not necessary to wash the flask in warm water as it should separate easily. The Ramitek lid is embedded in the top half of the flask.

Fig. 8-11

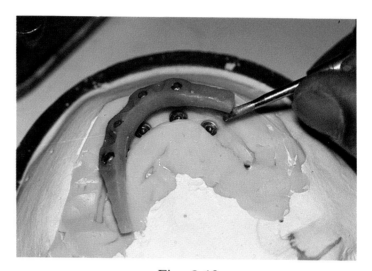

After making sure that the mold of Ramitek has the desired extension, the frame is unscrewed.

Fig. 8-12

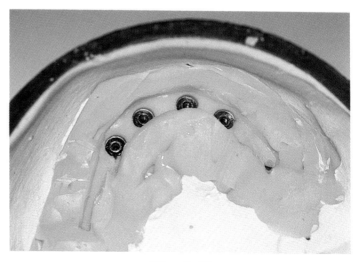

The titanium cylinders are removed from the acrylic frame and steam cleaned.

Fig. 8-13

They are mounted back to the master cast using clean 10.0 mm guide pins.

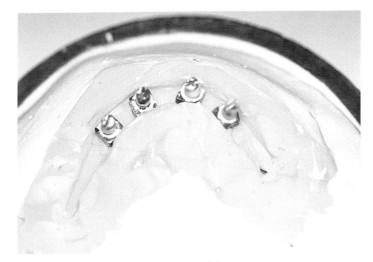

Fig. 8-14

A 1.5 mm to 2.0 mm layer of heat-polymerized acrylic (Lucitone 199, Dentsply Int.) is placed on the bottom of the Ramitek mold.

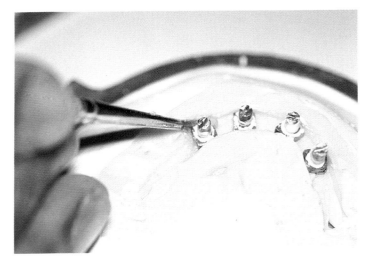

Fig. 8-15

Cut away approximately 0.5 centimeters of Ramitek at the distal ends to give a nice rounded effect.

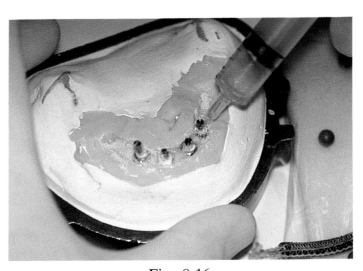

Fig. 8-16

It is now time to mix the resin for the bridge framework. Pour the activator powder into the acrylic container and stir for one minute. Leave the mixed acrylic for ten minutes (refrigerate if possible), or until all air bubbles have disappeared.

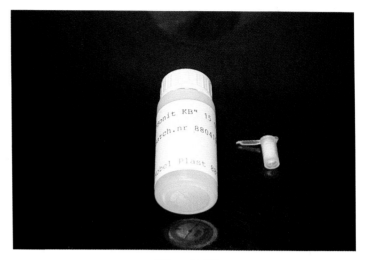

Fig. 8-17

A special syringe is filled by slowly drawing the acrylic mixture into it. When the syringe is filled, an injection needle is attached to its end. The needle is now screwed onto the fiber tube using a special nut.

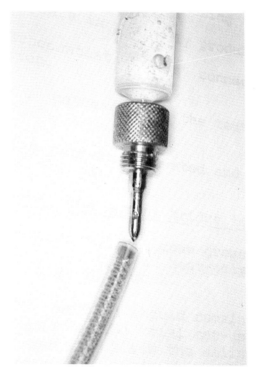

Fig. 8-18

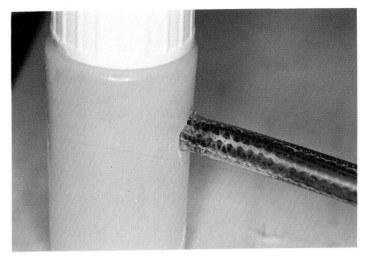

An empty plastic bottle is attached to the end of the tube for the purpose of collecting the surplus acrylic.

Fig. 8-19

Hold the fiber package, which is incorporated in a plastic tube, in a vertical position and slowly inject the mixed acrylic into the tube from underneath. This procedure takes about ten minutes to insure that the fiber is saturated and that all air is evacuated.

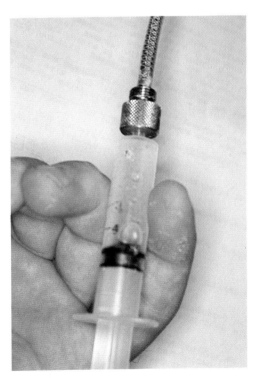

Fig. 8-20

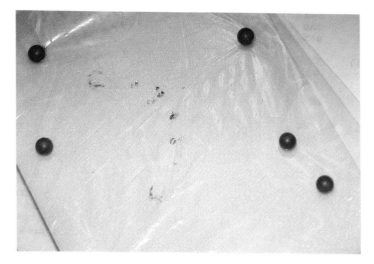

Cover the lower part of the flask with plastic foil and mark the positions of the titanium cylinders and the general outline of the frame to be with a felt tip pen. The plastic foil is then transferred in an upside down position to a piece of hard foam rubber and stretched flat using pins.

Fig. 8-21

The stainless steel transfer tip.

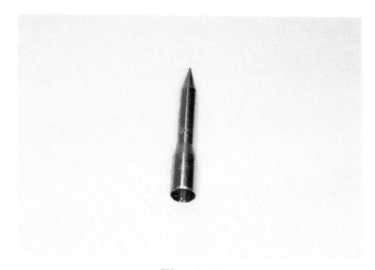

Fig. 8-22

Cut off the plastic covering of the fiber and starting at one end, mold and pin the carbon fiber on the plastic foil using the felt pen outline as a guide. Surplus acrylic is used to soak the fiber package while this procedure is done.

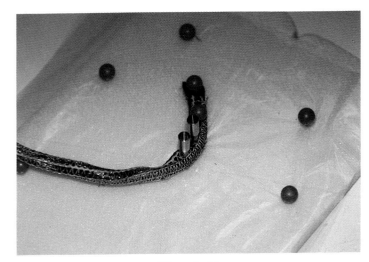

Fig. 8-23

Allow the stainless steel transfer tips to penetrate the fiber package at the marked abutment sites. Finally, the fiber package is cut to the desired distal extensions.

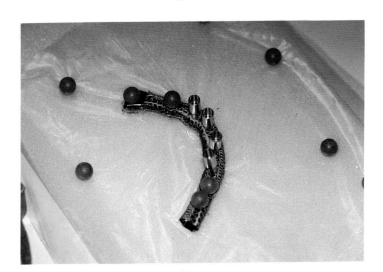

Fig. 8-24

More acrylic is injected onto the bottom of the framework mold and the secured titanium cylinders. The fiber package is then transferred from the foam rubber by lifting the plastic foil.

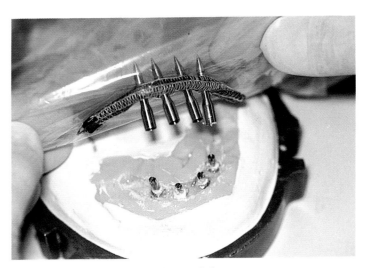

Fig. 8-25

Turn the plastic foil, uncured fiber, and transfer tips over; place the entire ensemble onto the titanium cylinders and press into place using forceps, a knife or tubing.

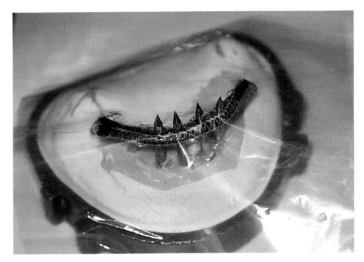

Fig. 8-26

Remove the plastic foil and fit the fiber package into the Ramitek void. To give the framework the desired shape, cut off pins are hammered into the plastic around the frame lingually, as well as buccally.

NOTE: The pins must not penetrate the fiber package.

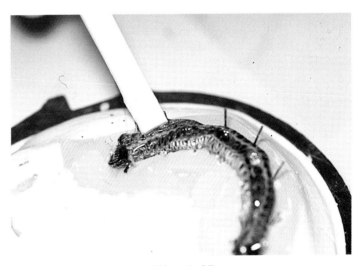

Fig. 8-27

Direct the pins inward when hammering so that the frame is given a high profile, while at the same time making room for the prosthesis acrylic buccally and lingually.

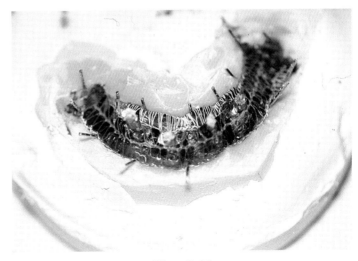

Fig. 8-28

When the framework has the desired profile, it may be necessary to cut one or more of the pins so as not to interfere with the plaster in the opposing half of the flask. The pins must not protrude more than the thickness of the Ramitek in the opposing half of the flask. Finally, the surplus acrylic is injected into both halves of the flask and the flask is closed. The frame is then cured for three hours at 80° C under 4 KG of pressure; then two hours at 98-100° C under the same pressure.

After the frame is cured and allowed to bench cool it is carefully broken out.

NOTE: Extra care must be taken when breaking out the frame. The master cast must be kept intact so that the matrix with teeth can be fitted to it and the master cast can be remounted on the articulator to verify the occlusion and placement of teeth.

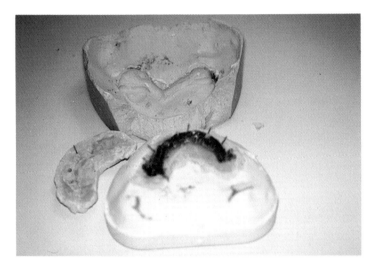

Fig. 8-29

After the master cast and frame are recovered, the black frame must be opaqued. For the sake of experimentation, and at the acceptance of the patient, three different opaques were used: 1) Dentacolor (Kulzer Co.); 2) D-Paque (Amco Co.); and 3) Lee Metal Primer (Lee Pharmaceutical). All opaques work well with the exception of a slight bleed-through of the D-Paque.

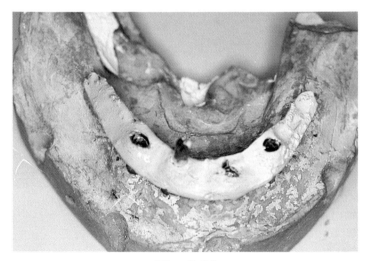

Fig. 8-30

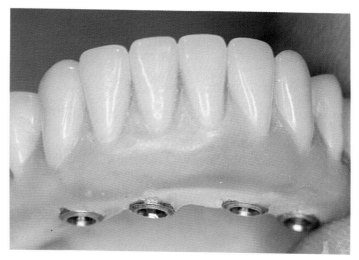

The teeth are now set on the frame and verified for fit and esthetics intraorally. A labial view of the carbon fiber frame with the teeth set and waxed to contour.

Fig. 8-31

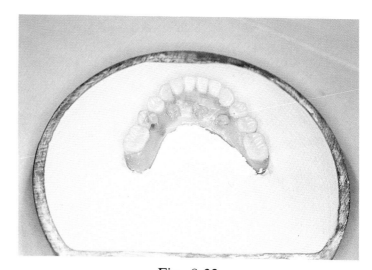

Guide pins are used to secure the brass replicas in the frame setup, and a processing model is fabricated (see Chapter 3). Screw slots are covered with Ramitek for easy recovery. The case is processed in Lucitone 199 for nine hours at 165° F.

Fig. 8-32

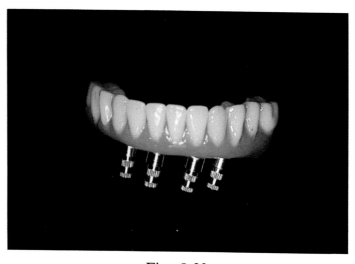

The prosthesis is finished, polished, and ready for insertion. A labial view illustrates good tissue color and adequate acrylic for proper lip support.

Fig. 8-33

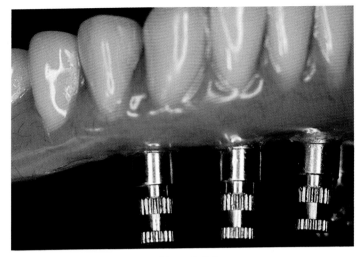

The correct use of opaque successfully masks the black graphite frame.

Fig. 8-34

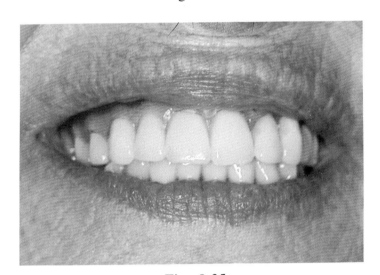

The finished prosthesis is placed intraorally, with function and esthetics restored.

Fig. 8-35

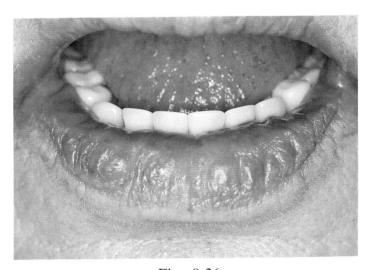

Good diagnostic treatment planning is evident with this carbon fiber-supported Tissue Integrated Prosthesis.

Fig. 8-36

Chapter 9

Resolving Esthetic Problems Created by Implant Alignment

The Double Casting Technique

The following patient treatment demonstrates one laboratory process used to overcome problems encountered when implants are aligned in unusual positions. These problems often become more apparent at the laboratory stage rather than in the clinical setting.

Laboratory design plan

It is evident in the framework's design stage that the fixture placement prevents a normal or traditional restorative approach. When the gold cylinders are placed on the brass replicas of the master cast, the guide pins protrude into the middle of the anterior teeth (Figs. 9-3 and 9-4). Continuing with the guide pins in this position destroys the labial surfaces of the teeth, creating an unacceptable esthetic result. Also, the patient's high lip line requires special placement of the cervix of the teeth in relation to the ridge mucosa. Denture teeth are selected and diagnostically set to evaluate esthetics (Fig. 9-5). When the diagnostic wax-up is completed, the framework design requires a double casting technique. This consists of an implant-retained substructure bar[1] securing an overcasting with screw and tube attachments (Fig. 9-6) (see Chapter 4). This design enables the castings to have both a firm anchor to the implants and to avoid screw access openings in the labial surfaces of the restorative teeth.

Method of fabrication

The substructure casting connecting the gold cylinders is constructed with plastic bars and DuraLay. The tube portion of the tube screw attachment is secured to the bar with DuraLay while being held parallel to the path of insertion. This path is determined by the incisal edge position and labial surface of the restorative teeth (Fig. 9-7). The path of insertion is also milled into the lingual and labial surfaces of the bar (Fig. 9-8). A labial tooth matrix is used here to determine the clearance available for the screw attachments (Fig. 9-9). When the tubes are positioned, the processing screws are lubricated and inserted. After final waxing, the bar is sprued, invested and cast with a Type IV gold alloy (T-IV-L, Nobelpharma). The bar is then carefully devested and all surfaces are finished (Fig. 9-10). The bar is steam cleaned and autoclave sterilized for a casting try-in (Fig. 9-11). Following a successful clinical try-in of the substructure bar, the overcasting is fabricated. The base or foundation for this pattern is an 0.3 mm thick plastic disc which is heated and vacuum formed over the substructure bar with a Dentsply Vacupress (Dentsply International). This produces superior results in the areas of stability and removal of the pattern. This pattern is carefully trimmed, and the end of each tube is exposed and the round ferrules luted to the pattern with self-cure resin.

Finally, retention rods and loops are attached and the pattern is coated with retentive beads (Fig. 9-12). The finish line between gold and acrylic is now carved in and formed into a bezel shape. A final check with the tooth matrix is helpful here to insure minimum bulk of the overcasting pattern. The pattern is then sprued up, invested, and cast using the same Type IV gold alloy used for the substructure (Fig. 9-13). After careful devesting and finishing, the overcasting is seated on the substructure and then rechecked with the tooth matrix for labial clearance (Fig. 9-14). Again cleaned and sterilized, both castings are tried in the mouth and checked radiographically for accuracy (Fig. 9-15). The teeth are then processed to the overcasting with a quality heat-cured acrylic (Hi-I, Fricke Dental Manufacturing). Following acrylic finishing and final polishing, the double casting screw-retained T.I.P. is prepared for delivery (Figs. 9-16 and 9-17).

The clinical appearance of the prosthesis shows one implant visible at its junction with the bridge. Also, the acrylic in the interproximal area does not match the surrounding mucosa. This condition frequently calls for the use of a Gingival Replacement Unit[2] (Figs. 9-18 and 9-19). Using the Gingival Replacement Unit to improve the esthetics of the prosthesis works very nicely. This small prosthesis is fabricated chairside using light-cured resin (Figs. 9-20 and 9-21).

This patient exhibits a partial edentulous area in the maxillary anterior area of teeth #'s 7, 8, 9, and 10.

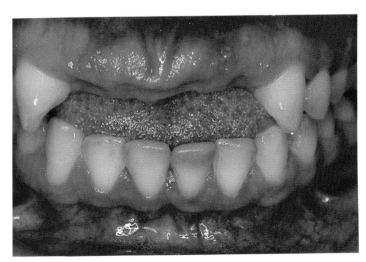

Fig. 9-1

Due to underlying bone structure, the two Brånemark implants cannot be surgically placed in the preferred position.

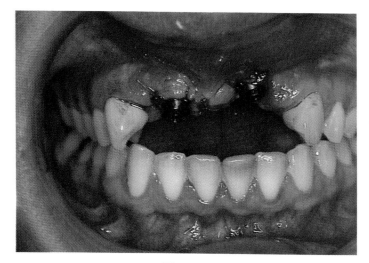

Fig. 9-2

This cross-arch view shows the relationship present between maxillary and mandibular anterior teeth in centric occlusion.

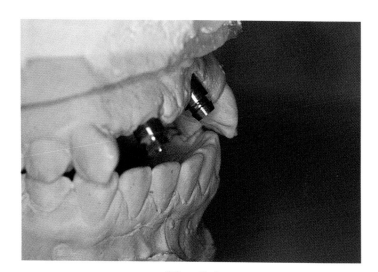

Fig. 9-3

A frontal view further demonstrates the difficult dimensions that must be overcome to achieve the desired esthetic result. The implant in the area of teeth #'s 7 and 8 is the most labial of the two. A smaller gold cylinder with a flathead screw is placed here to conserve interarch space.

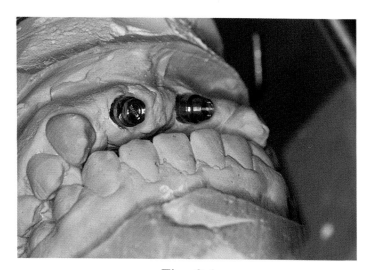

Fig. 9-4

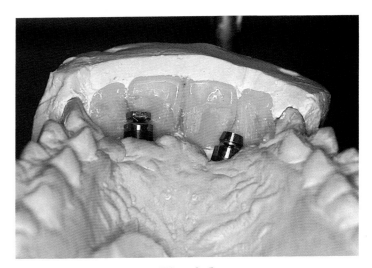

This lingual view shows the denture teeth held in position by a plaster matrix. Note the hollow areas cut into the teeth to create room for the prosthesis.

Fig. 9-5

Each component of the restoration is shown by this diagrammatic drawing.

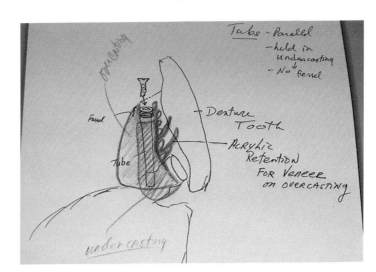

Fig. 9-6

A plastic bar is attached to the hard DuraLay rings with fresh resin. The tooth matrix is used here to help in the accurate placement of the bar.

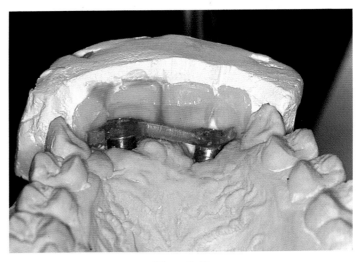

Fig. 9-7

The female tube attachment is positioned parallel to the desired path of insertion.

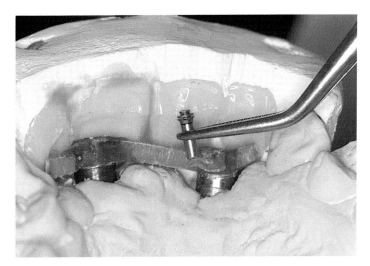

Fig. 9-8

Processing screws are placed in the fixed tubes and checked for clearance. The bar is then milled parallel on the lingual and labial surface.

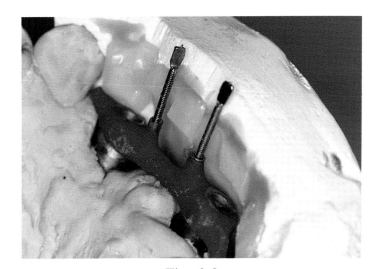

Fig. 9-9

An occlusal view of the finished substructure bar shows small distal cantilevers that improve the stability of the overcasting.

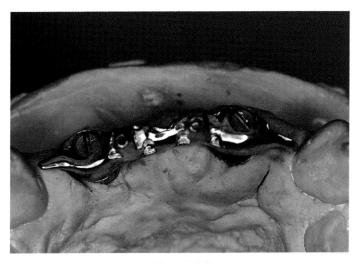

Fig. 9-10

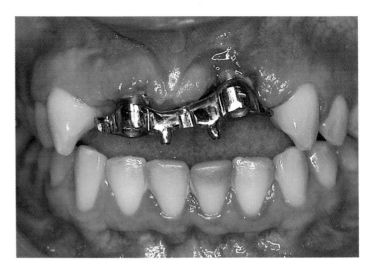

Notice the parallel walls and good marginal fit at the implant junction in this labial view of the clinical try-in of the substructure bar.

Fig. 9-11

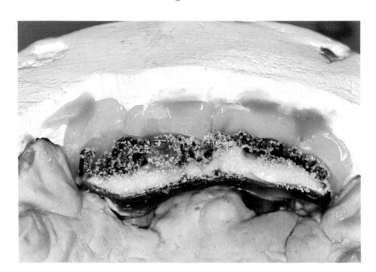

The finished overcasting pattern is checked for labial clearance with the tooth matrix.

Fig. 9-12

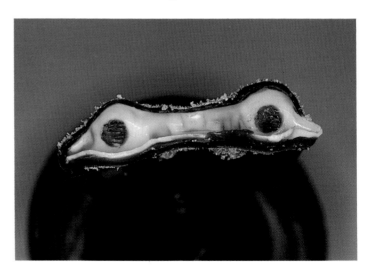

The internal portion of the pattern is shown here before the investing procedure.

Fig. 9-13

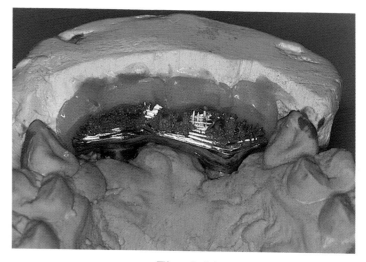

Both castings are seated on the master model and again tested for clearance with the tooth matrix.

Fig. 9-14

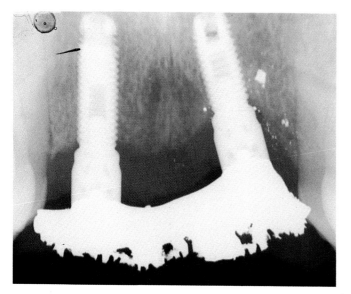

Both castings are tried intraorally and verified by radiograph for fit.

Fig. 9-15

The processed and finished prosthesis is shown in this labial view.

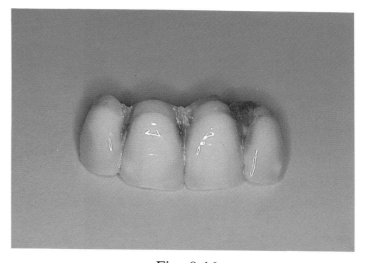

Fig. 9-16

Both castings are examined prior to packing and delivery.

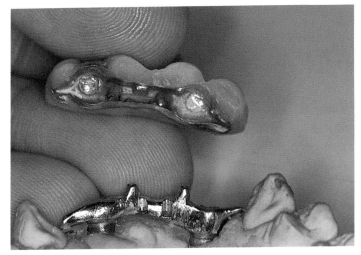

Fig. 9-17

A postoperative view of the patient with the prosthesis inserted.

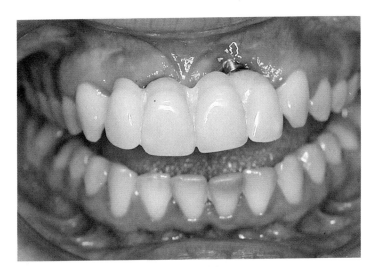

Fig. 9-18

The custom-fitted gingival replacement unit is light cured at chairside to insure accuracy.

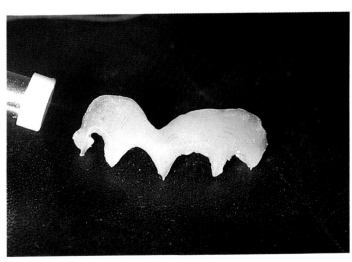

Fig. 9-19

Some slight finishing and polishing is done to perfect the Gingival Replacement Unit.

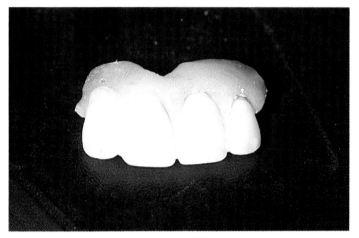

Fig. 9-20

With the entire prosthesis in place, a comparison with Figure 9-18 illustrates a dramatic improvement in esthetics created by the Gingival Replacement Unit.

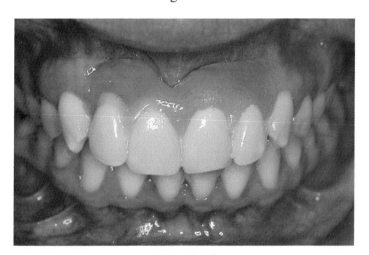

Fig. 9-21

The Brånemark System Angulated Abutment

The angulated abutment by Nobelpharma is a very innovative component designed to adjust access hole position, prosthetic screw angulation and improve cosmetics. This thirty-degree, twelve-sided, internal-designed component offers twelve different positions to drastically change the angulation of a severely misaligned implant.

Many times it is possible to determine the need for an angulated abutment at the time of second stage surgery (the abutment connection). It is also possible for the experienced technician to inform the clinician of the need for the angulated abutment after the casts are articulated.

Before the development of this abutment, if screws and access holes were positioned jutting through the labial aspect of an anterior tooth, there were basically three options: 1) the double casting technique as previously described; 2) unsightly patch marks which closed the access holes after final insertion; or 3) the combination of implant-supported posts securing a crown and bridge-type prosthesis.

The cast (Figure 9-25) described in this section presents with regular abutments in place at second stage surgery. After articulation (Figure 9-26), esthetic problems are evident.

A prosthesis is fabricated (Figure 9-27) with teeth flared and aligned in a manner to hide the access hole.

The angulated abutment with the abutment screw which screws directly into the internal threads of the implant is shown here.

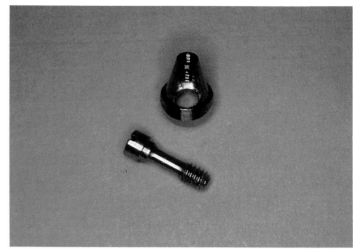

Fig. 9-22

The angulated abutment can be positioned twelve different ways. This is a view of the underside.

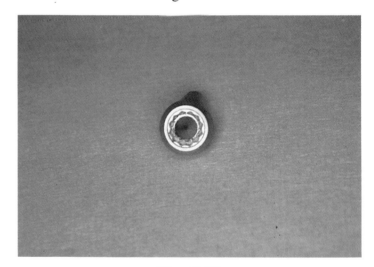

Fig. 9-23

The entire angulated system: implant, angulated abutment and abutment screw, gold cylinder and prosthetic screw, brass replica, impression piece, and healing abutment.

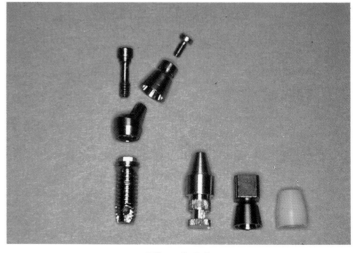

Fig. 9-24

This is the master cast, with regular abutments showing unfavorable labial inclination.

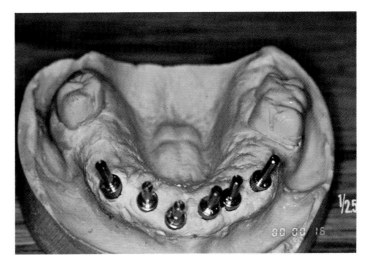

Fig. 9-25

As the casts are articulated, the unfavorable inclination becomes more evident.

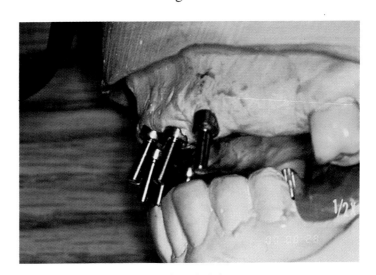

Fig. 9-26

An initial prosthesis was fabricated using the traditional hardware. Note the unsightly miscolored central incisor. The access hole in this tooth is filled with cold cure acrylic because the alignment of the implant caused the screw to protrude through the labial surface. After months of wear, the resin changed color, as many cold cure resins will do. A light-cured material can be used, but it is difficult to accurately match tooth shades.

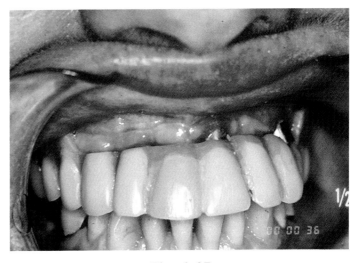

Fig. 9-27

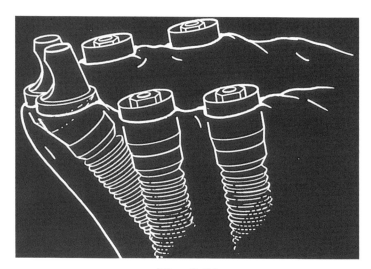

Fig. 9-28

These severely misaligned implants are drastically improved by use of the angulated abutment.

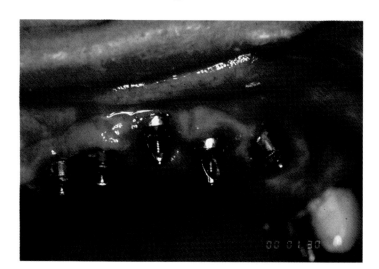

Fig. 9-29

Two angulated abutments are shown intraorally. Note the screw access hole that allows the use of a screwdriver to secure abutments to the implant.

Incisal view.

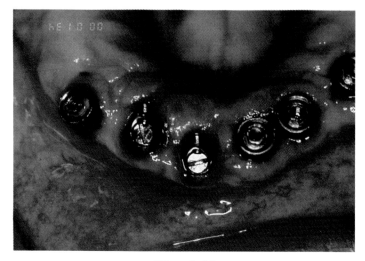

Fig. 9-30

The healing abutment is shown being attached to the angulated abutment and implant.

NOTE: The healing abutment is used as a precautionary device to inhibit tissue growth around the areas where the angulated cylinder will make contact in the finished prosthesis. This is used while the surrounding tissue heals and during fabrication of the prosthesis.

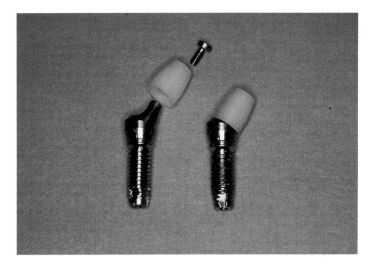

Fig. 9-31

The healing abutment is shown in place.

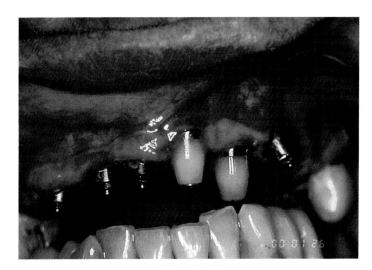

Fig. 9-32

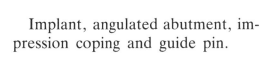Implant, angulated abutment, impression coping and guide pin.

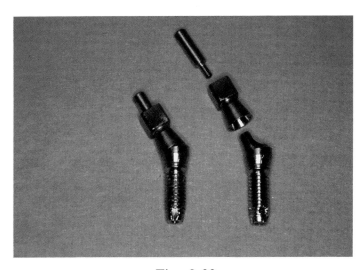

Fig. 9-33

This intraoral photo shows the impression copings in place. Compare the original articulated casts in Figure 9-26 with the angulated abutments to observe the drastic change in the angulation of the guide pins.

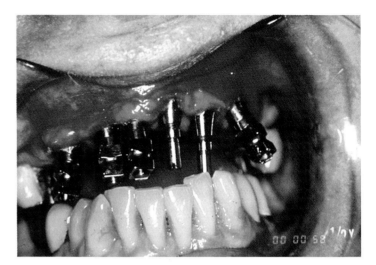

Fig. 9-34

The master impression shows good adaptation around the impression copings. It is now ready to have the brass replicas placed and the master cast poured.

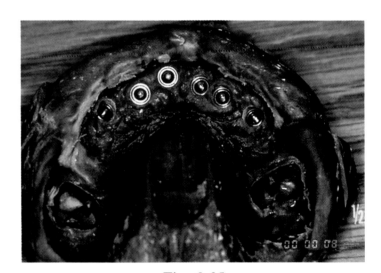

Fig. 9-35

Brass replicas for angulated abutment.

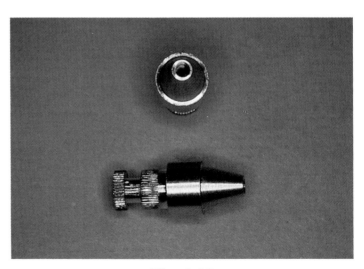

Fig. 9-36

The cast is poured with improved die stone.

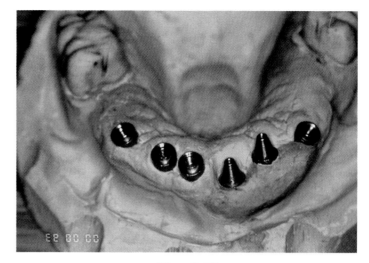

Fig. 9-37

The gold cylinders are in place.

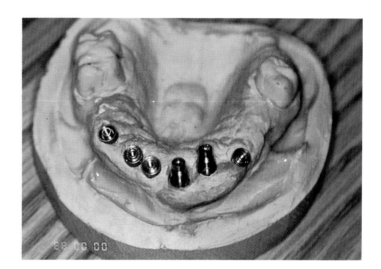

Fig. 9-38

The teeth are set in wax and tried in for esthetics, form, and function (see Chapter 3).

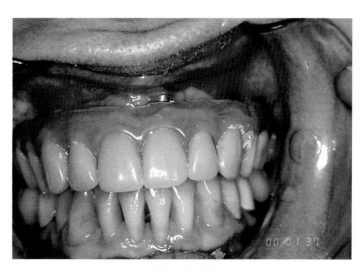

Fig. 9-39

The gold framework is waxed, cast, and verified intraorally and radiographically for fit. The teeth are set to frame and processed (see Chapter 3 for frame fabrication and denture processing).

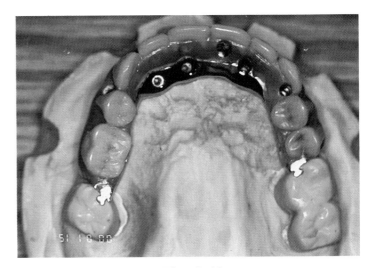

Fig. 9-40

The restoration is polished and ready for insertion.

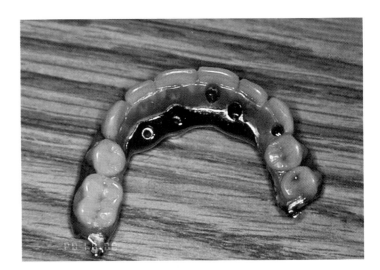

Fig. 9-41

This is a view of the underside of the restoration. It is very important that the gold framework be highly polished to reduce plaque buildup.

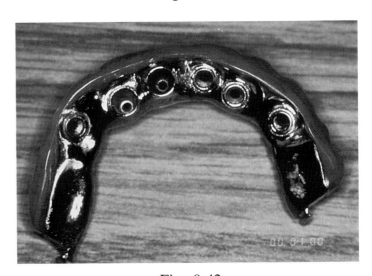

Fig. 9-42

The patient shows greatly improved esthetics, with all anterior access holes hidden to lingual of the prosthesis.

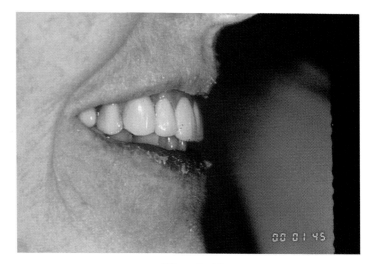

Fig. 9-43

Improved Access Hole Position With The Modified Core-Vent Screw Post Attachment

This maxillary cast shows six Core-Vent implant replicas. The long axis angulation of these implants presents a difficult situation in which to create the desired esthetic result.

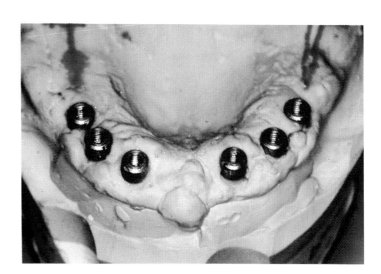

Fig. 9-44

An acrylic baseplate is fabricated using two plastic sleeves (Core-Vent #PSO) and Titanium fixation screws (Core-Vent #TSF). All undercuts are blocked out prior to the application of the clear acrylic (Orthocryl Caulk, Dentsply).

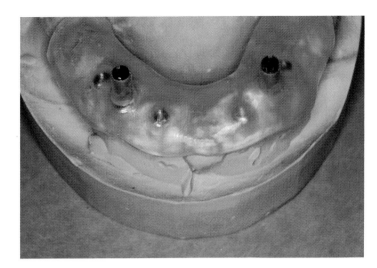

Fig. 9-45

With soft bite wax added to the acrylic base, the occlusal vertical dimension is established. The screw-retained bite rim offers added stability and increased accuracy to this procedure.

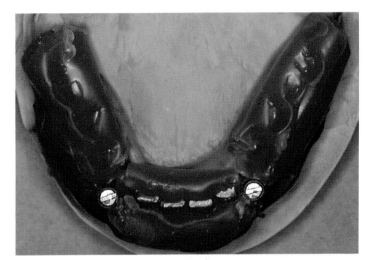

Fig. 9-46

The selected prosthetic teeth (Bioblend IPN, Dentsply) are set up in a Class I occlusal scheme. A duplicate clear acrylic baseplate is fabricated and used as a base for the wax setup. The setup is tried intraorally and checked for esthetics and occlusion.

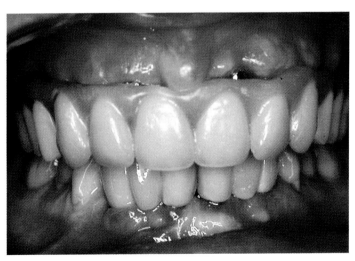

Fig. 9-47

An alginate impression is taken of the approved wax setup mounted to the master cast. A stone model is poured and prepared. A clear acetate vacuum-formed matrix is made. The matrix is refitted to the master cast using the palette as a guide. The diagnostic information provided by the clear matrix is crucial in determining the ultimate positions of the screw access holes.

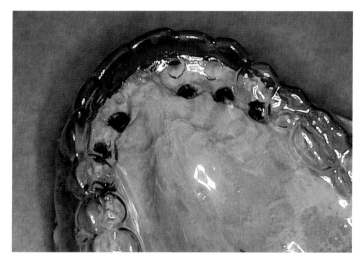

Fig. 9-48

The castable PC2 at right is shortened to the desired height, then hollowed out to accommodate the screw housing (Core-Vent #TSFH). The clear matrix will show the position of the angulated screw in relationship to the available lingual anatomy.

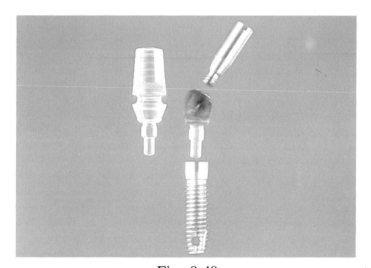

Fig. 9-49

A cross-sectional view reveals the internal screw threads, the female portion of the TSFH, and the modified PC2. This pattern is sprued up and invested using a high heat phosphorus material (Cermagold II, Whip Mix Corp). After the recommended burnout procedure, the ring is cast in (Palliag-M, Degussa Corp.) following the manufacturer's specifications. A special casting screw is provided for use during the casting procedures to preserve the integrity of the female screw heads.

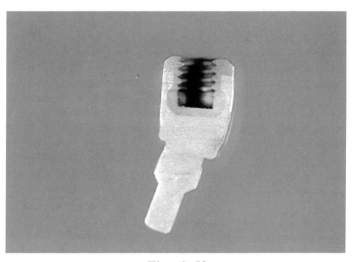

Fig. 9-50

The pattern is carefully devested and the casting screw removed. Maintaining the detail and condition of the post portion of this attachment is critical in the anti-rotational design of the implant component. All areas exposed to the oral cavity are highly polished.

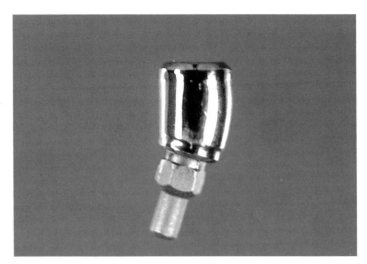

Fig. 9-51

This is the maxillary master cast with six finished screw posts and titanium fixation screws.

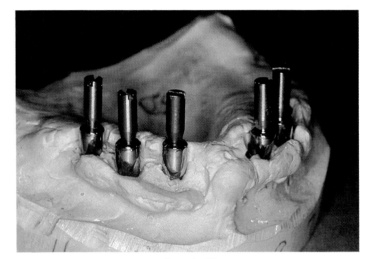

Fig. 9-52

The screw posts are tried in and verified for fit. Note the comparison of the soft tissue surrounding the implants with the stone reproduction in Figure 9-44.

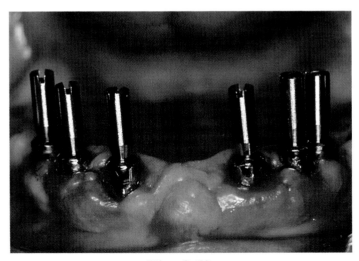

Fig. 9-53

The full intraoral view shows good screw angulation made possible by the modified screw post attachment.

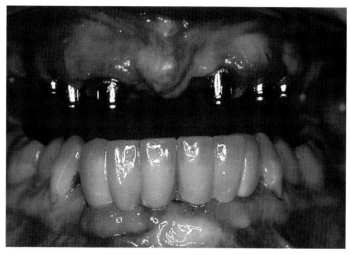

Fig. 9-54

A framework is designed using six castable plastic sleeves (Core-Vent #PSO) and six titanium fixation screws (Core-Vent TSF). This design is to accommodate a processed acrylic resin base with acrylic resin teeth (see Chapter 3). The frame pattern is checked with the matrix, sprued up, invested, and cast in (Palliag-M, Degussa Corp.) in the recommended manner. The castability of the Core-Vent sleeves permits the use of virtually any suitable metal. The casting is devested, cleaned, and all metal finishing completed. The accuracy of fit between the framework and the master cast must be completely passive.

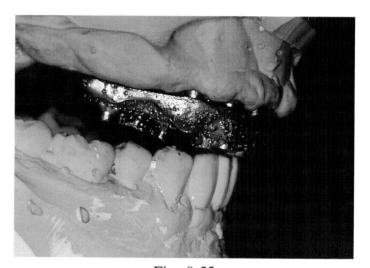

Fig. 9-55

The metal frame is tried in the mouth and checked for proper fit.

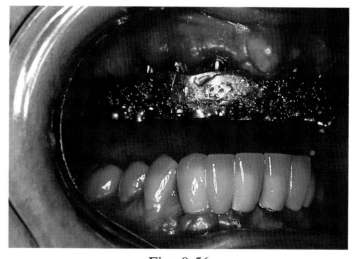

Fig. 9-56

The teeth are set in wax on the metal framework and verified again for esthetics. Setup is approved and the prosthesis is processed in Lucitone 199 (see Chapter 3). Esthetics are preserved with access holes lingual to all denture teeth through the use of the modified screw post attachment.

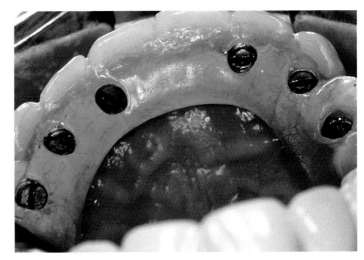

Fig. 9-57

With a thorough knowledge of available components and their use, it is possible to create an esthetic and functional prosthesis where misaligned implants are present.

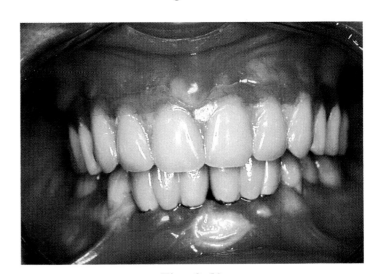

Fig. 9-58

References

1. Balshi T. Resolving esthetic complications using a double casting technique. *Quint Int.* 1986;17:281-287.
2. Balshi T, Parel S, Cardenas, Sullivan D. Gingival augmentation for osseointegrated implant prostheses. *J Pros Dent.* 1986;56:208-211.

Chapter 10

Guidelines for Problem Solving and Trouble Shooting

In working with implant-supported prostheses since 1982, many difficult and unusual problems have been encountered. The techniques that we have developed through our long-term experience can save time, experimentation, and frustration.

Even the most thorough planning and meticulous fabrication techniques can sometimes go awry. The creative technician can further develop and modify existing components and procedures to fit demanding situations.

Metal frameworks can fracture or be ill-fitting. Special soldering techniques are used to correct the alignment and integrity of fit between gold cylinders and titanium abutments.

Many times extreme masticatory forces are present in patients with implants.[1(pp. 271-2)] Since proprioception is lost, it is difficult for the patient to determine their biting forces.[1(pp. 89-97)] The result is prosthetic teeth being forced away from their position on the fixed denture bridge. The maxillary anterior lingual bite plate was developed for some patients as a solution to this problem.

The inability to remove laboratory guide pins from the processed denture bridge is another problem area. A heating implement is held on the threaded part of the embedded guide pin. As heat is transmitted, the acrylic in the immediate area of the guide pin will soften slightly and the guide pin can be forced through and removed (Fig. 10-19).

Pink porcelain can be used to esthetically enhance the restoration or to hide an unsightly gold cylinder.

An impression can be taken at the fixture level and the diagnostic cast used to determine the correct abutment. This technique can save chairside time, laboratory procedures and the cost of incorrect abutments.

Post Soldering A Ceramo-Metal Tissue-Integrated Prosthesis

The tissue-integrated prosthesis shown does not fit after the porcelain is baked to the framework and sectioned into two pieces.

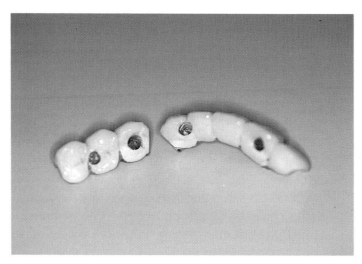

Fig. 10-1

Both sections are screwed into place and a plaster matrix is taken.

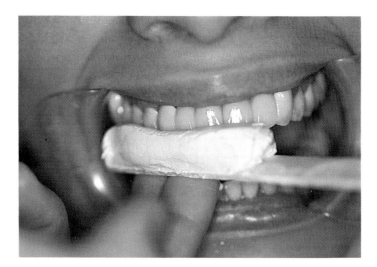

Fig. 10-2

Brass replicas are fastened to the gold cylinders with guide pins. The porcelain is blocked out with wax to eliminate contamination.

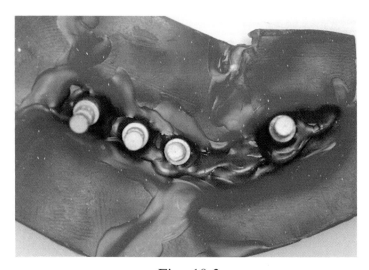

Fig. 10-3

This cross-section reveals the relationship of the matrix, bridge, wax block-out and brass replicas.

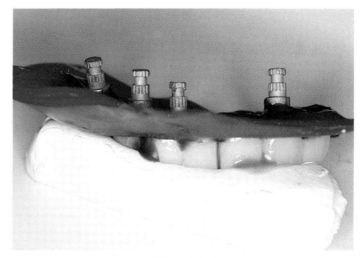

Fig. 10-4

The yellow stone cast is used to verify the accuracy of the soldering procedure.

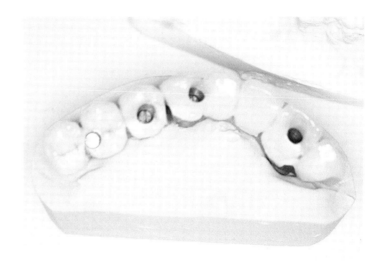

Fig. 10-5

Four Brånemark System titanium implants are used to stabilize the bridge in the investment. Special soldering replicas are now available.

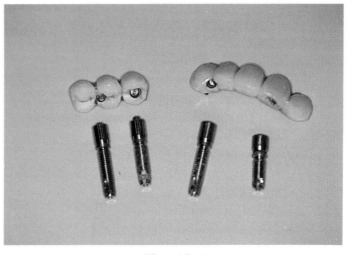

Fig. 10-6

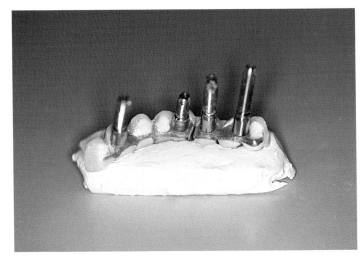

Fig. 10-7

After attaching the implants to the bridge, the matrix is used to check the fit.

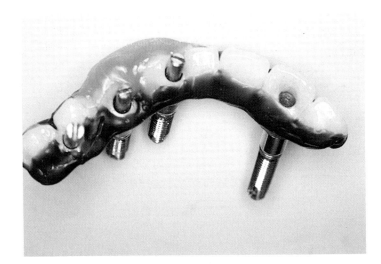

Fig. 10-8

After two sections are luted together, the porcelain is blocked out with wax.

High heat soldering investment (Whip Mix Corp.) is mixed according to the manufacturer's ratio and poured to form a firm base. Note how the porcelain is clean and free of any stone or investment. The model is placed in a cold burn-out oven and heated to 1,000°F. It is then placed in a porcelain oven and heated to 1,450°F. A high gold solder (Jelenko 615, Jelenko Co.) with a melting point of 1,365°F is then fluxed lightly and flowed into the joint. The model is then removed from the oven and bench cooled.

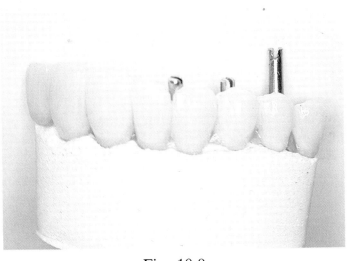

Fig. 10-9

After careful divesting, the solder joint is inspected. The metal is carefully polished using the protective replicas for the cylinders.

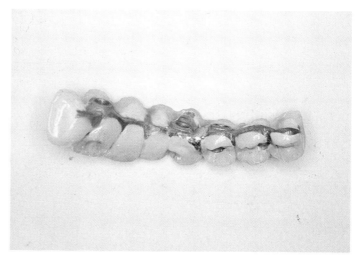

Fig. 10-10

This intraoral view illustrates excellent esthetics and fit.

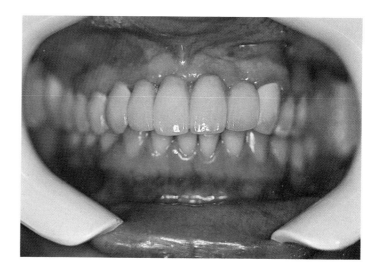

Fig. 10-11

The maxillary anterior lingual biteplate is used when a balanced occlusion cannot be attained. The lower teeth strike the gold framework instead of the pink acrylic and/or the prosthetic teeth. This greatly reduces the possibility of acrylic fractures and the "popping off" of teeth. This gold substructure maxillary frame with lingual biteplate is ready for tooth wax-up.

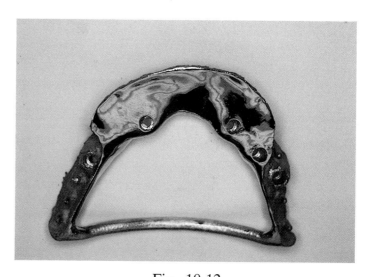

Fig. 10-12

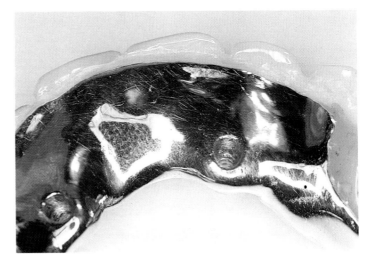

This is the finished prosthesis with anterior teeth securely luted to the frame.

Fig. 10-13

Because of the vertical opening, it is sometimes necessary to add pink porcelain to the prosthesis. Mixtures of different porcelain powders and modifiers are needed to attain the correct patient tissue color.[2] This gold substructure has pink opaque added to the tissue flanged area.

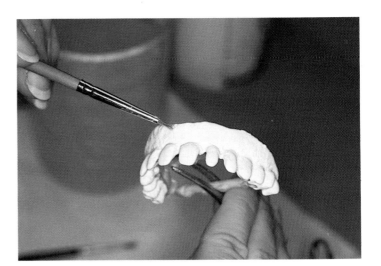

Fig. 10-14

The finished prosthesis ready for insertion. Note the fine detail at the cemento-enamel junction.

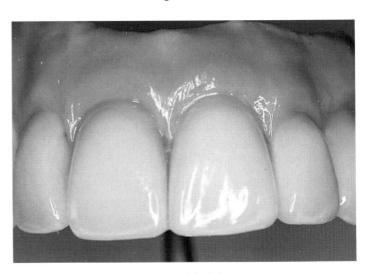

Fig. 10-15

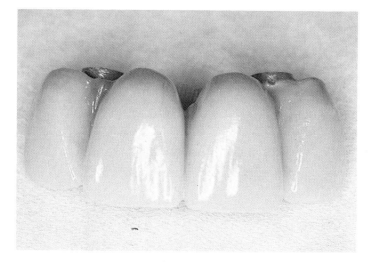

Pink porcelain is added interproximally to mask the underlying cylinders.

Fig. 10-16

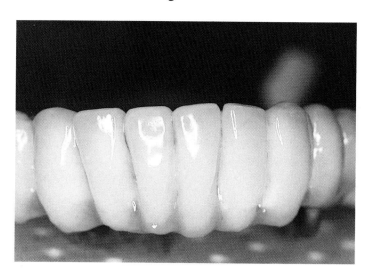

Sometimes small portions of pink porcelain are added to enhance the restoration esthetically.

Fig. 10-17

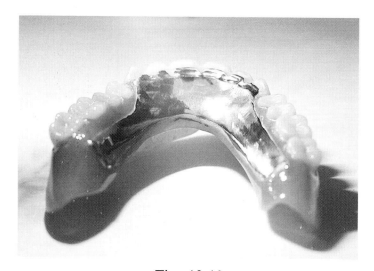

Because overdentures are hollowed out internally, their strength diminishing, it is sometimes necessary to cast a metal backbone to prevent breakage. This lingual view shows a finished maxillary overdenture with a metal backbone incorporated in acrylic. The underside of the frame has loops and beads to secure it to the acrylic. The tissue side of the prosthesis is all acrylic to enable the clinician to reline it as needed.

Fig. 10-18

A heating implement heats the gold screw and softens the surrounding acrylic for easy removal.

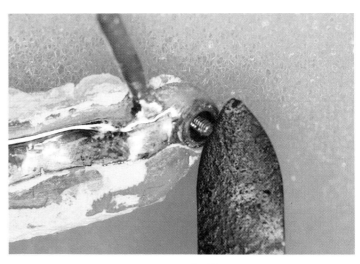

Fig. 10-19

Castable Telescopic Screw Attachment

The castable telescopic screw attachment (Preat Corporation) is a treatment plan alternative when only one implant is available for support. This eliminates the need for an occlusal opening that would accompany a standard key latch or tube and screw attachment. Since this is a castable pattern, any suitable metal may be used. This system may be used in conjunction with abutment telescopic copings. A minimum of 4.5 mm of vertical space from tissue to opposing tooth contact is required.

The abutment restoration is waxed to receive the male attachment. This male attachment is waxed directly over the crest of the ridge and in tissue contact.

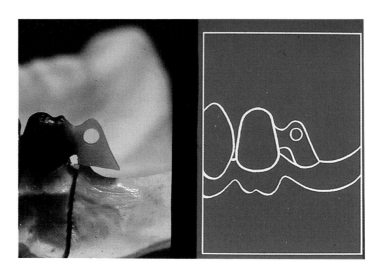

Fig. 10-20

The castable screw and abutment male attachment pattern are sprued, invested, and cast following the protocol described in Chapter 4. Devest the castings. Do not remove from the button. The male thread cleaner is used to refine the internal threads.

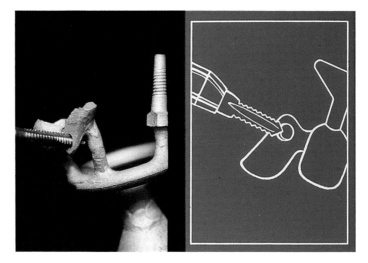

Fig. 10-21

The female thread cleaner must be used to refine the screw threads. Complete rubber wheeling and polishing of the shank portion of the screw before sectioning from the button.

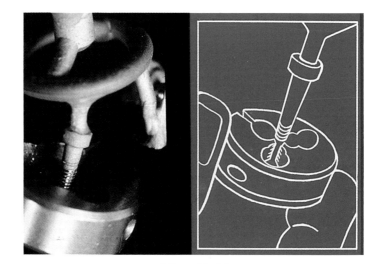

Fig. 10-22

The male attachment is polished and the crown portion is finished to receive the porcelain. The area of the Brånemark System abutment is indicated by the gold screw.

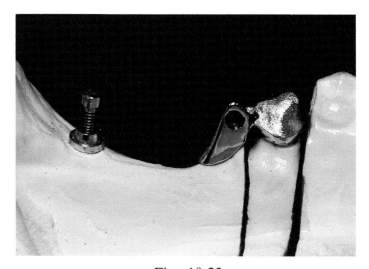

Fig. 10-23

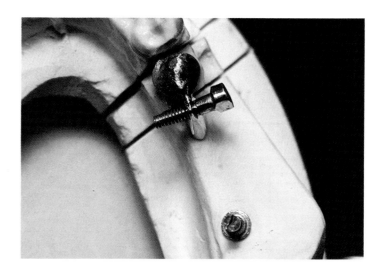

Lubricate the cast abutment restoration and the attachment male and screw. Thread the screw fully into the threaded recess with hand pressure.

Fig. 10-24

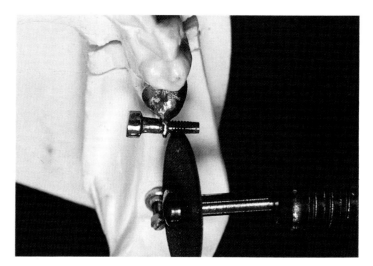

Back the screw out 1/4 turn. Cut off excess screw threads. It is recommended that the screw insert from the buccal side for easy access.

Fig. 10-25

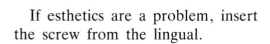
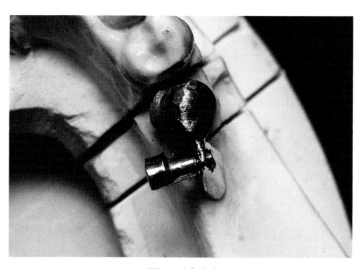

If esthetics are a problem, insert the screw from the lingual.

Fig. 10-26

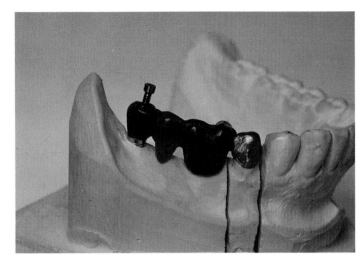

Fig. 10-27

The remaining portion of the substructure pattern is waxed around the screw and male attachment. The gold cylinder is screwed into place on the fixture replica and incorporated into the pontic wax-up.

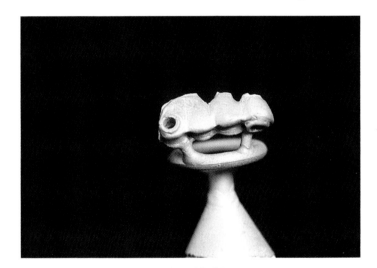

Fig. 10-28

The pattern is sprued, invested and cast.

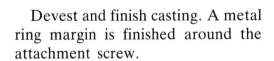

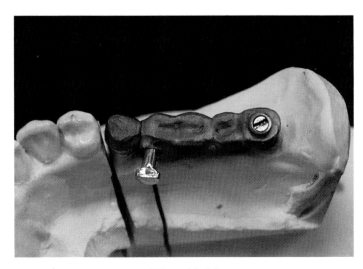

Fig. 10-29

Devest and finish casting. A metal ring margin is finished around the attachment screw.

The metal is cleaned, degassed, and opaqued. Gingival and incisal porcelains are blended, contoured and baked.

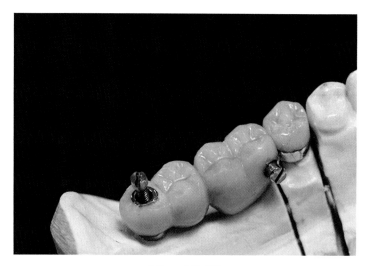

Fig. 10-30

The case is tried intraorally and all adjustments are made.

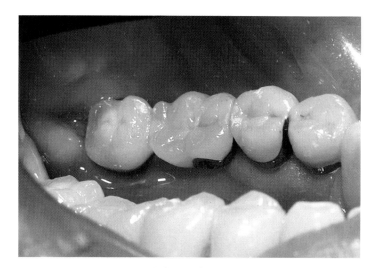

Fig. 10-31

A buccal view of the finished prosthesis. Note the proper occlusal anatomy without screw access hole filler or attachment hardware visible.

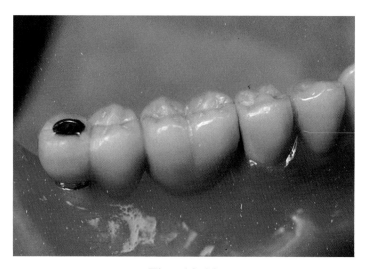

Fig. 10-32

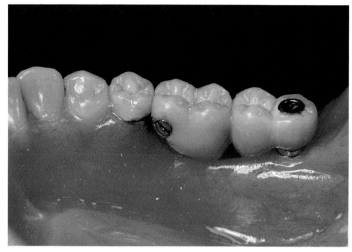

The lingual view illustrates good anatomical tooth contour incorporating the telescopic screw assembly.

Fig. 10-33

Full Arch Maxillary Temporary Splint

This full arch master impression incorporates natural tooth abutments, impression copings and all necessary soft tissue areas.[3]

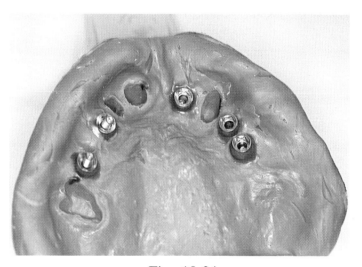

Fig. 10-34

Each coping is sealed lightly to the impression with wax (3-I Co. #ILA 20).

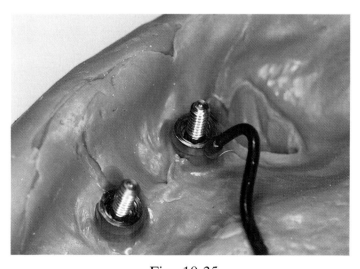

Fig. 10-35

The fixture replicas are screwed into place and the stone cast is poured.

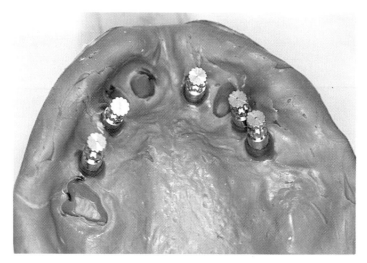

Fig. 10-36

The implant sites are numbered on the cast.

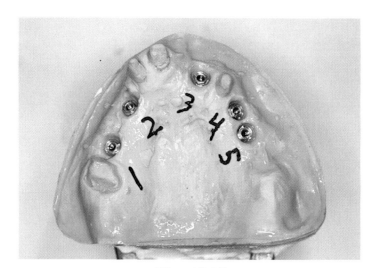

Fig. 10-37

The clear plastic stent is vacuum formed over the study cast of the patient's previous dentition. This stent is very valuable in determining tooth position, size and occlusal relationships.

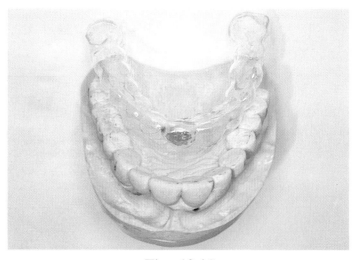

Fig. 10-38

Using the stent, the vertical dimension and midline are established.

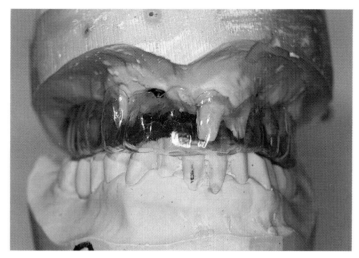

Fig. 10-39

Temporary metal cylinders and screws (3-I Co. #ITC 31) are used. The cylinders are adjusted individually to each fixture position for sufficient incisal clearance.

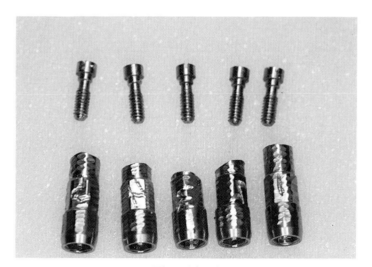

Fig. 10-40

Retention grooves are cut into the cylinders, along with the number matching the fixture position on the cast. A "3" is clearly visible on the surface of the cylinder.

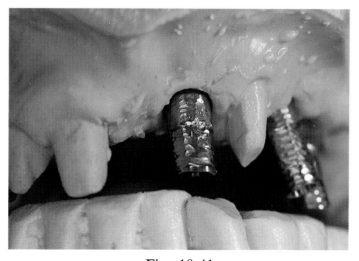

Fig. 10-41

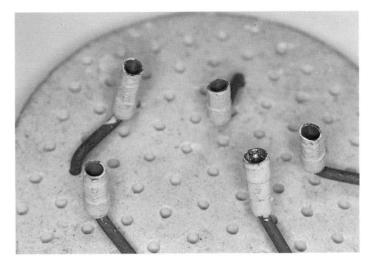

Fig. 10-42

All cylinders are sandblasted, ultrasonically cleaned and treated with light-cured opaque (Kulzer Co.).

The master cast is lubricated and all opaqued temporary cylinders are correctly placed numerically. Waxing procedures can now begin.

NOTE: If fixture placement and access hole position are not esthetic, problem solving abutments can now be selected. Using the articulated casts, we now have a gauge to determine proper abutment size and angulation. With this information, optimum results can be achieved in the final prosthesis.

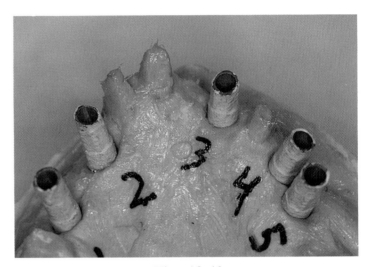

Fig. 10-43

Upon completion, the wax pattern is removed from the cast. The final contour and additions are made and the fixture replicas are fastened to the cylinders with laboratory guide pins. A processing model is poured as per protocol in Chapter 3. The case is invested in an arch form flask following normal techniques.

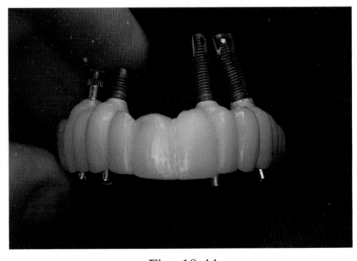

Fig. 10-44

The separated flask after boilout. Separating liquid is applied to stone areas in contact with the acrylic. Shade-matched acrylic (HI-I, Fricke Dental) is mixed to ratio, packed and pressed. After the gingival shade is cured, it is cut back from the incisal, interproximal and occlusal areas. A beveled slope is cut into the middle third of the teeth to mimic the characteristics of mesial inclination and gradual translucency.[4] Incisal acrylic is mixed, applied and pressed into place. The final curing stage is now initiated.

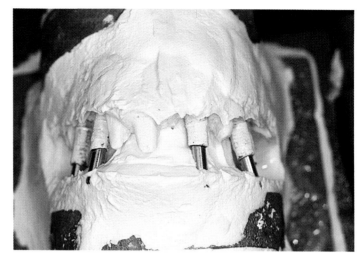

Fig. 10-45

After curing, careful devesting procedures should be employed.

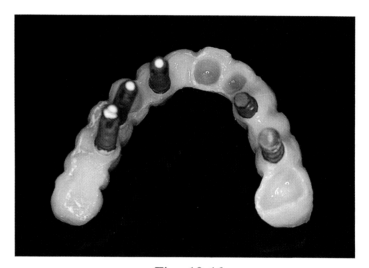

Fig. 10-46

The fulcrum created by the long laboratory screws and fixture replicas can easily fracture the prosthesis. All hardware should be removed prior to finishing the acrylic.

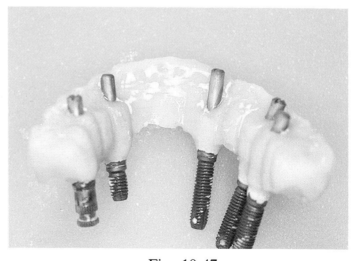

Fig. 10-47

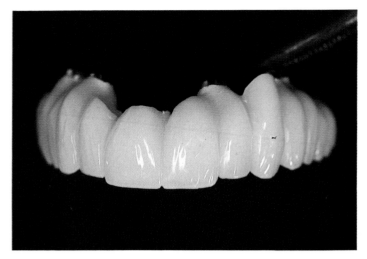

This view shows the full-arch acrylic temporary after contouring and final polishing. Extensive buccal-labial tooth root development produces a correct emergence profile. The residual ridge resorption requires this modification to provide adequate cheek and lip support.

Fig. 10-48

Partial Edentulous Mandibular Denture Format Temporary

When a conversion prosthesis is not available, it is sometimes necessary to fabricate a short-term denture format implant-supported acrylic T.I.P. This will only serve as an interim device until the final prosthesis can be made.

Cylinders are screwed into place and blocked out (see Chapter 3). Cold cure acrylic is mixed, molded around the cylinders and an acrylic bridge formed to encompass the edentulous areas. A metal reinforcement should be incorporated in the lingual aspect of the prosthesis for strength, especially in the cantilever area. After curing, the acrylic frame and model are steam cleaned. The frame is shaped and smoothed with acrylic finishing burs. The frame should be at least 3-4 mm in width and as high as the prosthesis will allow.

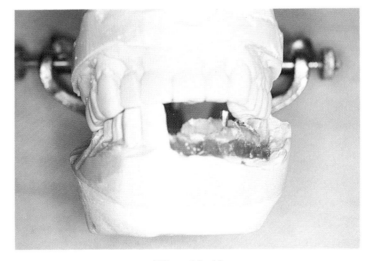

Fig. 10-49

The denture teeth are then selected.

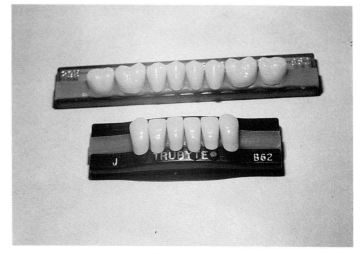

Fig. 10-50

The denture teeth are set and waxed to contour.

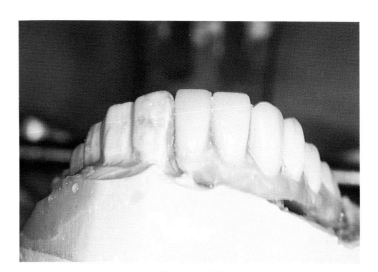

Fig. 10-51

The denture bridge is removed from the cast and the brass replicas are secured with guide pins. A processing model is fabricated (see Chapter 3).

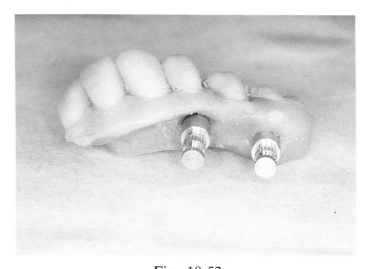

Fig. 10-52

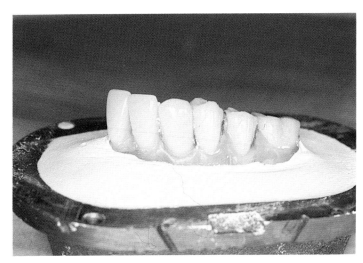

The prosthesis is flasked in the conventional manner.

Fig. 10-53

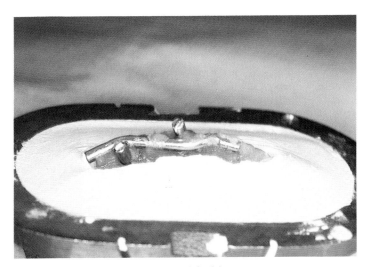

The prosthesis is boiled out and all stone areas are painted with a separating medium. Note that the metal bar runs the entire length of the T.I.P. The flask is packed using Lucitone 199 and cured for 9 hours at 165° F.

Fig. 10-54

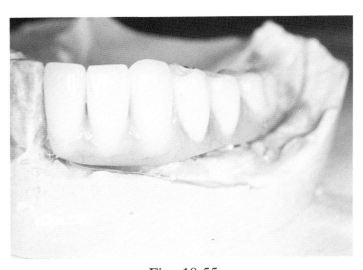

After curing, the restoration is broken out, cleaned, finished, and polished.

Fig. 10-55

References

1. Zarb GA, Jansson T. In: Brånemark P-I, Zarb GA, Albrektsson T, eds. *Tissue Integrated Prostheses: Osseointegration in Clinical Dentistry*. Chicago: Quintessence Publishing Company; 1985.

2. Cook PA, Girswald WH, Post AC. The effect of superficial colorant and glaze on the surface texture of vacuum-fired porcelain. *J Prosthet Dent*. 1984;51:476-484.

3. Sullivan DY. Prosthetic considerations for the utilization of osseointegrated fixtures in the partially edentulous arch. *Int J Ral and Maxil Imp*. 1986;1:39-46.

4. Mumford G. Recent studies in porcelain crown construction. Paper read before Partial Prosthodontics Section, American Dental Association, Philadelphia, Penn., October 1961.

Chapter 11

A Look to the Future

There are many new frontiers that await the dental technician who looks to the future. New techniques, applications, and materials in the implant field which have been clinically tested will soon be available. Among these are the implant-supported extraoral prostheses: eyes, noses, ears, and joints. In addition, computer-assisted machinery for the fabrication of dental prostheses (CAD-CAM) is a reality that must also be addressed by the progressive dental technician.

New component and abutment designs are being developed rapidly. The complete dental technician will keep abreast of new information concerning progressive implant hardware and be able to successfully integrate the new technology into his laboratory.

Figures 11-1 through 11-6 illustrate one example of maxillofacial reconstruction accomplished with the aid of endosseous implants. Patients who otherwise would have been adversely affected both physically and psychologically can now lead a relatively normal life. (Photographs courtesy of Dr. P.J. Henry)

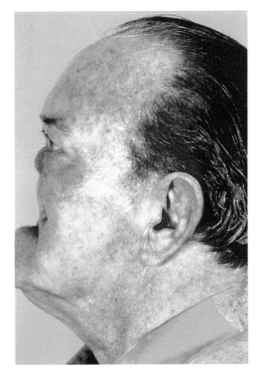

Fig. 11-1

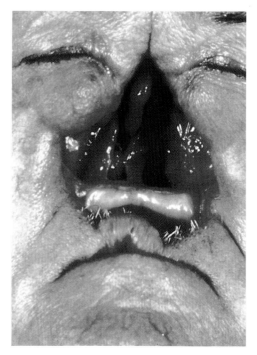

Fig. 11-2

Photographs courtesy of Dr. P.J. Henry.

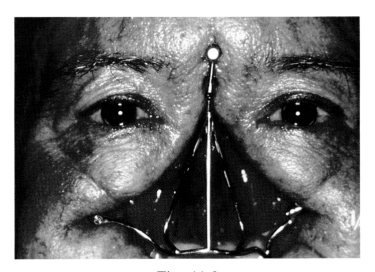

Fig. 11-3

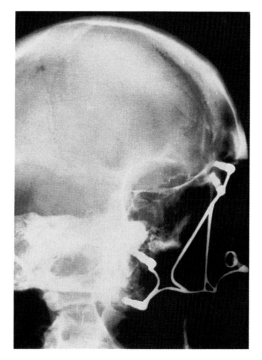

Fig. 11-4

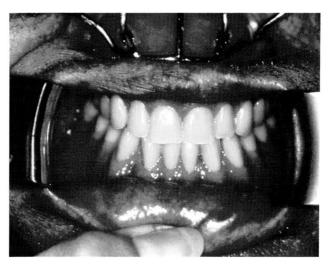

Photograph courtesy of Dr. P.J. Henry.

Fig. 11-5

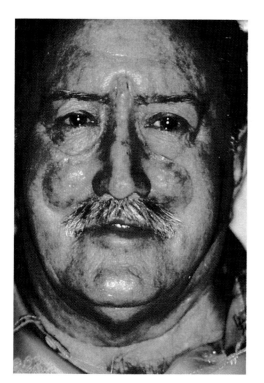

Photograph courtesy of Dr. P.J. Henry.

Fig. 11-6

CAD-CAM Technology

Computer Aided Design (CAD) and Computer Aided Manufacturing (CAM) represent a fascinating combination of art and science. One system that is currently on the market is the Procera™ System by Nobelpharma. Commercially pure titanium is used because of its unsurpassed biological properties and high degree of tensile strength. This system uses prefabricated cantilevers which are laser welded together to produce a perfectly passive fitting framework.

An additional benefit of the Procera System is that it can be used with either the traditional denture acrylic format or the ceramo-metal technique with the newly developed TICERAM™ porcelain.

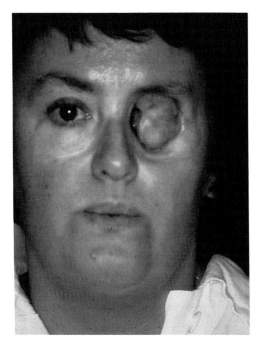

Fig. 11-7

Figures 11-7 through 11-11 illustrate the benefits of osseointegrated fixtures in the orbital region. A screw-retained bar with magnetic keepers will securely hold this facial prosthesis and eliminate the need for adhesives.[1]

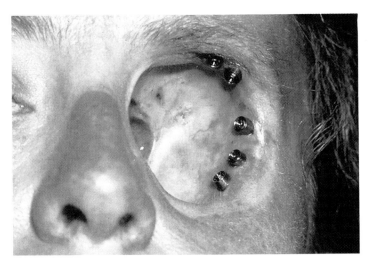

Fig. 11-8

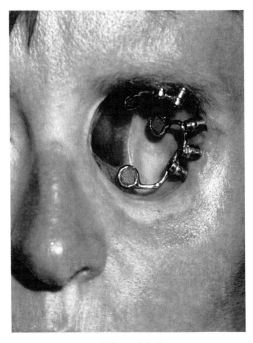

Fig. 11-9

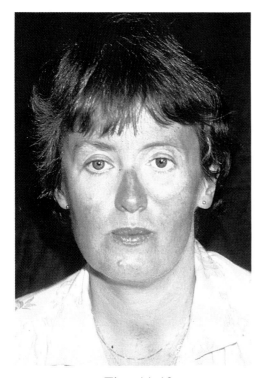
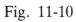

Fig. 11-10

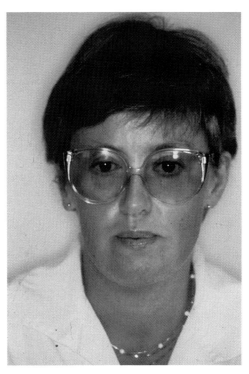

Fig. 11-11

This computer-controlled milling machine duplicates exactly the forms required for the titanium framework. (Figs 11-12 and 11-13)

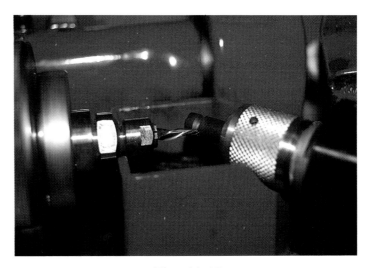

Fig. 11-12

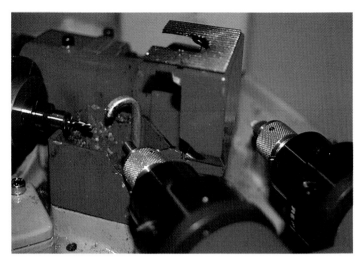

Fig. 11-13

After the titanium cantilevers are correctly positioned, they are brought to the laser welding machine for final connection. The laser welding machine has video monitors for quality control.

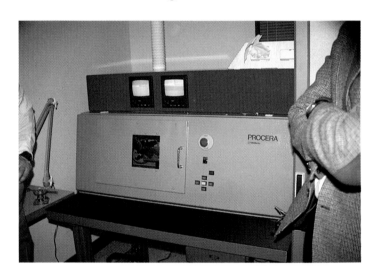

Fig. 11-14

An inside view of the welding chamber with blue laser welding arms at the center and black video lenses to either side.

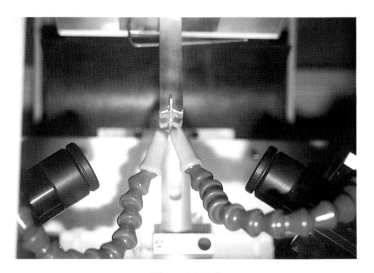

Fig. 11-15

References

1. Parel M and Tjellstrom A. The United States and Swedish experience with osseointegration and facial prosthesis. *Int J Oral Maxillofac.* 1991;6:75-79.

Manufacturers Listing

Accurate Set Incorporated; Newark, New Jersey
Amco Company; Philadelphia, Pennsylvania
Coe Incorporated; Chicago, Illinois
Coltene Incorporated; Hudson, Massachusetts
Degussa Corporation; Long Island, New York
Dentsply International; York, Pennsylvania
Espe Incorporated; Germany
Fricke Dental Manufacturing; Villa Park, Illinois
J.M. Ney Company; Bloomfield, Connecticut
Jelenko Company; Armonk, New York
Jeneric-Pentron; Wallingford, New York
Kerr Company; Promulus, Michigan
Kulzer Company; Werheim, Germany
L.D. Caulk; Milford, Delaware
Lee Pharmaceutical; South El Monte, California
Mizzy Incorporated; Cherry Hill, New Jersey
Nobelpharma USA; Chicago, Illinois
Parkel; Farmingdale, New York
Preat Corporation; San Mateo, California
Taub Products Company; Jersey City, New Jersey
Vita Zahnfabrik; Georgia
Whaledent International; New York, New York
Whip Mix Company; Louisville, Kentucky
William Company; Amherst, New York